Diagnosis and Management of Parkinson's Disease

Y0-CDE-975

Fifth Edition

Cheryl H. Waters, MD, FRCPC

Albert and Judith Glickman Professor
Department of Neurology
Columbia University Medical Center

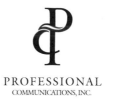

PROFESSIONAL
COMMUNICATIONS, INC.

Professional Communications, Inc.

A Medical Publishing Company

Marketing Office:	*Editorial Office:*
400 Center Bay Drive	PO Box 10
West Islip, NY 11795	Caddo, OK 74729-0010
(t) 631/661-2852	(t) 580/367-9838
(f) 631/661-2167	(f) 580/367-9989

For orders only, please call
1-800-337-9838
or visit our website at
www.pcibooks.com

ISBN: 1-932610-20-0

Printed in the United States of America

DISCLAIMER

The opinions expressed in this publication reflect those of the author. However, the author makes no warranty regarding the contents of the publication. The protocols described herein are general and may not apply to a specific patient. Any product mentioned in this publication should be taken in accordance with the prescribing information provided by the manufacturer.

This text is printed on recycled paper.

DEDICATION

This book is dedicated to my supportive husband, Paul; my four wonderful children, Stephanie, Richard, Jesse, and Sam; and my brave and devoted patients.

TABLE OF CONTENTS

TABLES

FIGURES

Introduction

The clinical management of the 1 million Americans afflicted with Parkinson's disease is poised to undergo major changes based on recent advances in pharmacologic and surgical therapy that promise significant improvement in patients' quality of life. Many of the new products and procedures are already available and others are in development or clinical trial. Among them are:

- A range of new and novel dopaminergic agents
- Methods of altering the administration, delivery, absorption, and metabolism of levodopa
- The possibility of neuroprotective therapy
- The potential manipulation of other neurotransmitter systems
- Novel surgical therapies
- New molecular biological neuroconstructive procedures and operative techniques that use gene therapy.

Thus the future looks optimistic for the maintenance of Parkinson's disease patients within the mainstream despite the need for continuing search for cause and cure of the disease.

The Diagnosis and Management of Parkinson's Disease has been prepared for physicians as a review of the etiology, pathophysiology, differential diagnosis, treatment, and management of Parkinson's disease. The author wishes to thank the investigators and clinicians whose experience and publications have supplemented her own as an investigator of the new pharmacologic therapies and made possible this up-to-date presentation of their applicability, efficacy, and nuances.

— *Cheryl H. Waters, MD, FRCPC*

1 Definition and Classification

Parkinson's disease (PD) is the most prevalent type of parkinsonism, a clinical syndrome caused by lesions in the basal ganglia, predominantly in the substantia nigra, that produce deficits in motor behavior.

Parkinsonism is a clinical rather than an etiologic entity since it is associated with several pathologic processes that damage the extrapyramidal system. Its many causes are divided into four categories (**Table 1.1**):

- Primary, or idiopathic (PD)
- Secondary parkinsonism (associated with infectious agents, drugs, toxins, vascular disease, trauma, brain neoplasm)
- Parkinson-plus syndromes
- Heredodegenerative diseases.

Parkinson's Disease

Parkinson's disease makes up approximately 80% of cases of parkinsonism.[1] The syndrome was first cogently described by James Parkinson in 1817 and named paralysis agitans by Marshall Hall in 1841.[2] Both description and label stress reduction in muscle power unduly, however, omitting rigidity and slowness of movement (akinesia), crucial to the characteristic tetrad known as TRAP:

- Resting **T**remor
- Cogwheel **R**igidity
- Bradykinesia/**A**kinesia
- **P**ostural reflex impairment.

Of this tetrad, only resting tremor is truly suggestive of PD, an early sign that may remain prominent

TABLE 1.1 — Classification of Parkinsonism

Idiopathic Parkinsonism
- Parkinson's disease, juvenile parkinsonism

Secondary Parkinsonism
- Drug-induced:
  - Dopamine receptor blockers (neuroleptics)
  - Dopamine depleters (reserpine, tetrabenazine)
  - Lithium
  - Flunarizine, cinnarizine, diltiazem
- Hemiatrophy-hemiparkinsonism
- Hydrocephalus:
  - Normal-pressure hydrocephalus
  - Noncommunicating hydrocephalus
- Hypoxia
- Infectious:
  - Fungal infections
  - AIDS
  - Intracytoplasmic hyaline inclusion disease
  - Subacute sclerosing panencephalitis
  - Postencephalitic
  - Creutzfeldt-Jakob disease
- Metabolic:
  - Hypocalcemic parkinsonism
  - Chronic hepatocerebral degeneration
- Paraneoplastic parkinsonism
- Psychogenic
- Syringomesencephalia
- Trauma
- Toxin:
  - MPTP intoxication
  - Carbon monoxide intoxication
  - Manganese intoxication
  - Cyanide
  - Methanol
  - Carbon disulfide intoxication
  - Disulfiram
- Tumor
- Vascular:
  - Multi-infarct
  - Binswanger's disease

Continued

Parkinson-Plus Syndromes
- Corticobasal degeneration
- Dementia syndrome:
  - Alzheimer's disease
  - Dementia with Lewy bodies (DLB)
  - Pick's disease
- Lytico-Bodig (Guamanian PD-D-ALS)
- Multiple system atrophy syndromes:
  - Striatonigral degeneration
  - Shy-Drager syndrome
  - Sporadic olivopontocerebellar atrophy
  - Motor neuron disease-Parkinson
- Progressive pallidal atrophy
- Progressive supranuclear palsy

Heredodegenerative Diseases
- Ceroid-lipofuscinosis
- Gerstmann-Sträussler-Scheinker disease
- Pantothenate kinase associated neurodegeneration (PKAN)
- Huntington's disease
- Lubag (Filipino X-linked dystonia-parkinson)
- Machado-Joseph disease
- Mitochondrial cytopathies with striatal necrosis
- Neuroacanthocytosis
- Familial olivopontocerebellar atrophy
- Thalamic dementia syndrome
- Wilson's disease

Abbreviations: AIDS, acquired immunodeficiency syndrome; MPTP, 1-methyl-4-phenyl-1,2,3,6-tetrahydropyridine; PD-D-ALS, Parkinson's disease-dementia-amyotrophic lateral sclerosis.

even late in the disorder.[2] The others occur in varying degrees in other forms of parkinsonism.

Secondary Parkinsonism

■ Postencephalitic Parkinsonism

Many patients who survived the acute febrile illness and encephalopathy during the 1919-to-1926 pandemics of encephalitis lethargica (von Economo's encephalitis) later developed a variety of movement disorders, including parkinsonism.[1] Although the virus(es) that caused the disease was never isolated, parkinsonism is associated with Coxsackie, Japanese B, and western equine encephalitis viruses. The underlying lesion in postencephalitic parkinsonism, depletion of the pigmented, dopamine-secreting neurons in an area of the substantia nigra, is similar to that of PD, but the former has a long latency after exposure to acute illness (a phenomenon not yet understood).

■ **Drug-Induced Parkinsonism**

A syndrome clinically indistinguishable from PD can be caused by drugs that:
- Deplete the synaptic stores of dopamine (reserpine, tetrabenazine)
- Block the dopamine receptors (antipsychotics and antiemetics)
- Cause selective destruction of the dopamine nigrostriatal pathway (the street drug contaminant methylphenyltetrahydropyridine [MPTP]).

■ **Pugilistic Encephalopathy**

Although some studies suggest that patients with PD may have had a higher incidence of significant head injuries with loss of consciousness than matched controls, others argue against the causative role of trauma.[3,4]

The widespread neurological dysfunction seen in the chronic traumatic encephalopathy of "punch-drunk" boxers may include some signs and symptoms of advanced PD, such as:
- Personality changes
- Memory impairment
- Dysarthria
- Tremor
- Ataxia.[3]

This "pugilistic dementia," unlike PD, is caused by severe blows to the brain stem and rotational torques, probably resulting in a series of microhemorrhages.

Parkinson-Plus

Patients with Parkinson-plus carry other features not associated with PD, including:[1,4]

- Supranuclear gaze palsy (progressive supranuclear palsy)
- Dysautonomia (multiple-system atrophy, Shy-Drager syndrome)
- Laryngeal stridor (striatonigral degeneration)
- Apraxia, myoclonus, and alien hand (corticobasal degeneration)
- Dementia syndrome (Alzheimer's disease, Lewy body disease)
- Amyotrophic lateral sclerosis (Lytico-Bodig, Guamanian Parkinson's disease-dementia-amyotrophic lateral sclerosis [PD-D-ALS]).

Heredodegenerative Parkinsonism

Inherited degenerative disorders include:

- Wilson's disease (a disease of copper metabolism)
- Huntington's disease
- Pantothenate kinase associated neurodegeneration (PKAN)
- Familial basal ganglia calcification
- Familial olivopontocerebellar atrophy.

REFERENCES

1. Jankovic J. The extrapyramidal disorders. In: Bennett JC, Plum F, eds. *Cecil Textbook of Medicine.* 20th ed. Philadelphia, Pa: WB Saunders Co; 1996:2042-2046.

2. Adams RD, Victor M, Ropper AH. *Principles of Neurology.* 6th ed. New York: McGraw-Hill; 1997:1067-1078.

3. Davie CA, Pirtosek Z, Barker GJ, Kingsley DP, Miller PH, Lees AJ. Magnetic resonance spectroscopic study of parkinsonism related to boxing. *J Neurol Neurosurg Psychiatry.* 1995;58:688-691.

4. Riley DE. Secondary parkinsonism. In: Jankovic J, Tolosa E, eds. *Parkinson's Disease and Movement Disorders.* 3rd ed. Baltimore, Md: Lippincott–Williams and Wilkins; 1998:317-340.

2 Epidemiology

As a rule, Parkinson's disease (PD) begins between the ages of 40 and 70, with peak age at onset occurring in the sixth decade. Onset at younger than age 20 is known as juvenile parkinsonism, which has a different pattern of nigral degeneration and is often hereditary (parkin gene) or caused by Huntington's or Wilson's disease. PD is more common in men, with a male-to-female ratio of 3:2.[1]

Parkinson's disease makes up approximately 80% of cases of parkinsonism. In North America, there are approximately 1 million PD patients; about 1% of the population over the age of 65 is afflicted.[1] The prevalence of PD is approximately 160 cases per 100,000 population, and the incidence is about 20 cases per 100,000 population.[1] But both prevalence and incidence increase with age: at age 70, they reach approximately 55 and 120 cases per 100,000 population per year, respectively.[1]

The incidence in all countries where vital statistics are kept is the same. Considering this frequency, coincidence in a family on the basis of chance occurrence might be as high as 5%.

REFERENCES

1. Goldman SM, Tanner C. Etiology of Parkinson's disease. In: Jankovic J, Tolosa E, eds. *Parkinson's Disease and Movement Disorders*. 3rd ed. Baltimore, Md: Lippincott–Williams and Wilkins; 1998:133-158.

3 Natural History

The pathological changes of Parkinson's disease (PD) may appear as much as 3 decades before the appearance of clinical signs. Onset is so gradual and insidious, however, that patients rarely can pinpoint the first symptom(s). Early symptoms may be so mild that a clinical diagnosis is not possible.

According to some patients, symptoms appeared only during periods of stress, then subsided only to reappear several years later.[1] Others describe a history of disability consistent with parkinsonism that was present many years before a definite diagnosis was made. Patients' families often recall subtle motor and mental changes that antedate the diagnosis by years.

A large body of evidence indicates the progression of PD may be rapid in the preclinical stage as well as during the first years of the disease, with subsequent slowing of the process.[2] According to the Deprenyl and Tocopherol Antioxidative Therapy of Parkinsonism (DATATOP) Unified Parkinson's Disease Rating Scale Study, motor examination scores declined at a rate of 8% to 9% per year in untreated patients.[3]

Before the introduction of levodopa, PD caused severe disability in 16% of patients within 5 years of onset, in 37% during the next 5 years, and in 42% of those surviving for 15 years.[4] The mortality rate continues to be higher than that in the general population matched for age, sex, and racial origin[5] in spite of numerous advances in pharmacological management.[6]

Once established, PD can follow several distinct clinical patterns. For example, two symptom-based subgroups have been noted: one dominated by postural instability and gait difficulty, a second by tremor.[7] Distinguishing features of the tremor group include:

- A family history of tremor
- Earlier age at onset
- Less functional impairment
- Preservation of mental status.

A later study questioned the more benign nature of "tremor-dominant" disease; however, in a follow-up study of 125 *de novo* PD patients (98 reassessed in 5 years),[8] a positive association was indeed found between *severity* of tremor and older age, dementia, and rapid progression of disability. But the definition of tremor dominant is unclear and varies in different studies, including its presence as initial symptom, chief complaint, or as only cause of disability, with no or minor rigidity or akinesia. The later findings confirm other reports that tremor is often less marked in the younger-onset patients, whose disease often follows a benign course.

Tremor is not always present at the onset of PD, however. It occurs more commonly in patients with early-onset (at age 40 and younger) disease, whereas postural instability and gait difficulty are more dominant in patients with late-onset (at age 70 and older).

The presence or absence of dementia underlies another possible classification.[9] The percentage of patients in whom the symptom develops is controversial, ranging from 10% to 41% in a number of studies.[9]

A third classification is based on the tempo of the disease: a benign form, found in 15% of patients, and malignant disease, with marked deterioration after a year of therapy. Finally, younger patients seem to experience a slower rate of progression but are much more troubled with motor fluctuations than are their older counterparts.

REFERENCES

1. Koller WC, Montgomery EB. Issues in the early diagnosis of Parkinson's disease. *Neurology*. 1997;49(1 suppl 1):S10-S25.

2. Poewe WH, Wenning GK. The natural history of Parkinson's disease. *Neurology*. 1996;47(6 suppl 3):S146-S152.

3. The Parkinson Study Group. Effect of deprenyl on the progression of disability in early Parkinson's disease. *N Engl J Med*. 1989;321:1364-1371.

4. Fahn S. Parkinsonism. In: Rowland LP, ed. *Merritt's Textbook of Neurology*. 9th ed. Baltimore, Md: Lea and Febiger; 1995:713-730.

5. Louis ED, Marder K, Cote L, Tang M, Mayeux R. Mortality from Parkinson disease. *Arch Neurol*. 1997;54:260-264.

6. Hely MA, Morris JG, Traficante R, Reid WG, O'Sullivan DJ, Williamson PM. The Sydney multicentre study of Parkinson's disease: progression and mortality at 10 years. *J Neurol Neurosurg Psychiatry*. 1999;67:300-307.

7. Jankovic J, McDermott M, Carter J, et al. Variable expression of Parkinson's disease: a base-line analysis of the DATATOP cohort. The Parkinson Study Group. *Neurology*. 1990;40:1529-1534.

8. Hely MA, Morris JG, Reid WG, et al. Age at onset: the major determinant of outcome in Parkinson's disease. *Acta Neurol Scand*. 1995;92:455-463.

9. Mindham RH. The place of dementia in Parkinson's disease: a methodologic saga. *Adv Neurol*. 1999;80:403-408.

4   Etiology

The cause of Parkinson's disease (PD), a subject rich in theories, probably is multifactorial, with contributions of variable significance from hereditary predisposition, environmental toxins, and aging. The probable contribution of endogenously generated toxic molecules is discussed in Chapter 5, *Pathophysiology*.

Aging

The fact that PD is one of the most common causes of disability among the elderly engendered two theories:

- That the disease is an accelerated form of aging
- That some acute exogenous or endogenous insult to the substantia nigra, followed by slow age-related nigral cell attrition, leads to the onset and progression of symptoms with increasing frequency after the sixth decade.

A characteristic histologic sign of PD, the presence of Lewy bodies in the substantia nigra, appears occasionally in aging nonparkinsonian individuals, perhaps as a herald of the disease had they lived long enough.[1] An autopsy series from the Baltimore Longitudinal Study of Aging found that α-synuclein lesions characteristic of PD and other α-synucleinopathies (see Chapter 6, *Pathogenesis*) were found in 100% of brains of PD patients but in only 8.3% of brains of normal elderly individuals.[2] Thal and colleagues looked at the pathologic changes characteristic of PD, Alzheimer's disease (AD), and dementia with Lewy bodies (DLB) in the brains of nondemented, asymptomatic, otherwise healthy elderly people. He was trying to determine if these changes represent the early stages of PD, AD, or DLB or the normal concomitants of aging.[3] The authors conclude that while aging is a major risk factor for these neurodegenerative diseases, it is not an inevitable cause.

Nigral cells have been shown to diminish normally with age, from about 425,000 to 200,000 by age 80 years. In PD, however, the overall number of pigmented neurons in the substantia nigra has been found to be reduced to about 31% of that in age-matched controls.

The pathological process of PD occurs predominantly in the relatively lightly pigmented neurons of the ventrointermediate and ventrolateral regions of the substantia nigra pars compacta, whereas age-related attrition is more often seen in the dorsal tier and pars lateralis, where neuronal melanin content is somewhat greater.[4]

Thus the speed of regional neuronal loss in aging is far less than that seen in PD and occurs in an area opposite that involved in PD.

While aging may not be a fundamental cause of PD, advanced age appears to be a contributing differentiating factor for certain clinical characteristics. Levy and coworkers assessed the contribution of aging to the severity of different motor signs in PD.[5] They found that axial (gait and postural) impairment in PD may result from the combined effect of the disease and the aging process. Another study compared the clinical presentation of PD patients with old-age onset ($\geq$78 years) with those with middle-age onset (between 43 and 66 years).[6] At a comparable length of PD duration (5.1 years and 5.6 years), the UPDRS motor score was significantly higher in those with old-age onset. Specifically, old-age onset patients had significantly higher scores for rigidity, bradykinesia, axial impairment, but not for tremor.

24

Genetics

There is much interest in the genetics of PD and the hope of one day finding the genetic and environmental factors that presumably cause PD. A seminal study of twins was undertaken to determine the relative importance of genetics.[7] Using a twin registry of World War II veterans, 20,000 surviving men were identified. Of those, 193 men were found to have PD. When these subjects were analyzed, there was virtually no heritability in those in whom the disease began after the age of 50. However, the four monozygotic twin pairs who were under the age of 50 at disease onset were all concordant for the disease.

The cause of PD in the majority of PD patients is probably multifactorial, resulting from the interaction of a number of genetic and environmental risk factors. Researchers have shown in a community-based study that the lifetime risk of PD in a parent or a sibling of an individual with PD is approximately 2%; this compares with a lifetime risk of PD of 1% in a parent or sibling of an individual who does not have PD.[8]

To date, six genes have been found to be associated with PD, mostly in a few rare, "PD families." In addition, we know the approximate locations of an additional four genes. Further research will uncover these genes and elucidate their role in the development of PD. The genes and loci are summarized in **Table 4**.1.

Of all of the genes discovered to date, the Parkin gene has been the most investigated. Mutations in this gene have been identified in a significant number of young-onset PD (YOPD) patients (≤50 years of age at onset) and families. The probability of finding mutations in this gene in individuals with YOPD has been found to decrease dramatically in those in whom onset occurs after age 30.[9] Mutations in Parkin are thought to account for approximately 18% of people with YOPD and no family history of PD and are also asso-

TABLE 4.1 — Genes and Their Loci Associated With Parkinson's Disease

Name/Gene Symbol	Location	Inheritance	Ethnic population	Reference
Alpha Synuclein SNCA/PARK 1/ PARK 4	4q21	Autosomal Dominant	Western Europe, Spellman-Meunter kindred – Iowa	Polymeropoulos et al[1] Farrer et al[2] Singleton et al[3]
Parkin /PARK 2	6q25.2-q27	Autosomal recessive/ susceptibility factor	Panethnic	Kitada et al[4]
PARK 3	2p13 (gene not localized)	Autosomal Dominant	Western Europe	Gasser et al[5]
Ubiquitin C-terminal esterase L1/PARK 5	4p14	Autosomal Dominant	Western Europe	Leroy et al[6]
PTEN-induced putative kinase 1/PARK 6	1p36	Autosomal Recessive	Panethnic	Valente et al[7]
DJ-1/PARK 7	1p36	Autosomal Recessive	Western Europe	Bonifati et al[8]
LRRK2/Dardarin/ PARK 8	12q12	Autosomal Dominant	Western Europe	Paisan-Ruiz et al[9]

Kufor-Rakeb syndrome/ PARK 9	1p36 (gene not localized)	Autosomal recessive	Jordan	Hampshire et al[10]
PARK 10	1p32 (gene not localized)	Late-onset susceptibility factor	Iceland	Hicks et al[11]
PARK 11	2q36-q37 (gene not localized)	Susceptibility factor	Panethnic	Pankratz et al[12]

1. Polymeropoulos MH, et al. *Science*. 1997;276:2045-2047.
2. Farrer M, et al. *Hum Mol Genet*. 1999;8:81-85.
3. Singleton AB, et al. *Science*. 2003;302:841.
4. Kitada T, et al. *Nature*. 1998;392:605-608.
5. Gasser T, et al. *Nat Genet*. 1998;18:262-265.
6. Leroy E, et al. *Nature*. 1998;395:451-452.
7. Valente EM, et al. *Science*. 2004;304:1158-1160.
8. Bonifati V, et al. *Science*. 2003;299:256-259.
9. Paisan-Ruiz C, et al. *Neuron*. 2004;44:595-600.
10. Hampshire DJ, et al. *J Med Genet*. 2001;38:680-682.
11. Hicks AA, et al. *Ann Neurol*. 2002;52:549-555.
12. Pankratz N, et al, for the Parkinson Study Group. *Am J Hum Genet*. 2003;72:1053-1057.

4

ciated with sustained response to levodopa and early occurrence of levodopa-induced dyskinesias, which are often severe. However, the Parkin-associated phenotype is broad and some cases are indistinguishable from idiopathic PD.

More recently, a single mutation in dardarin (PARK8), now known as LRRK2 (Leucine-Rich Repeat Kinase 2) has been discovered.[10] Mutations in the LRRK2 gene are of particular interest because they appear to be the most common mutations thus far identified in either familial or "sporadic" PD. The LRRK2 G2019S mutation alone has been reported in 2.8% to 6.6% of autosomal dominant PD families[11-13] and in 2% to 8% of sporadic cases.[14-16] The G2019S mutation has variable penetrance, with 17% at 50 years and 85% at 70 years, a profile that mimics idiopathic sporadic PD. This mutation appears to be common in the Ashkenazi Jewish population; out of 120 unrelated Ashkenazi Jewish patients with PD, 22 (18.3%) had this mutation.[17] Although other LRRK2 mutations are described, the G2019S mutation remains the most common mutation in patients with either sporadic or familial PD. This mutation has not been seen in Alzheimer's disease or in parkinsonian syndromes other than idiopathic PD.[18,19]

In general, the reported cases of LRRK2 mutations have typical features of PD with asymmetric onset of tremor, bradykinesia, and rigidity. As noted above, the age of onset is variable and occasionally is very late,[13] with one report of a carrier male reaching 89 years with only subtle neurologic changes.[20] Patients have a good response to levodopa but develop motor complications, including dyskinesias. Imaging using fluorodopa and PET, as well as ligands for the dopamine transporter with SPECT, demonstrate changes typical of those seen in idiopathic PD.[21]

Although researchers still have not discovered the genetic risk factors associated with most cases of PD, identification of genes involved in familial PD and YOPD hopefully will lead to an understanding of the cause of PD and to better diagnosis and treatment.

Environment

The theory that exposure to some exogenous agent may be the cause of PD was the result of the accidental intoxication of drug users by methylphenyltetrahydropyridine (MPTP), a contaminant in illicit street drugs. Patients presented with a sudden onset of all the symptoms of PD, although with less tremor and more cognitive and emotional disability, drooling, and gait and balance difficulty. Furthermore, the pathologic change characteristic of PD, the Lewy body, is not seen in experimental parkinsonism induced in primates by MPTP. Although clinical progression of MPTP-induced parkinsonism is rare, delayed-onset movement disorders have been reported in patients after transient exposure.[1]

Despite these clinical and pathological differences between the MPTP-induced condition and idiopathic PD, the use of MPTP in monkeys has provided an excellent animal model of the disease.

Actually, MPTP itself is nontoxic; rather, its oxidation product, 1-methyl-4-phenylpyridinium ion (MPP^+) is the culprit, found to be highly destructive to neurons containing melanin pigment, such as those in the substantia nigra. MPTP is oxidized to MPP^+ by monoamine oxidase type B (MAO-B), one of the isoenzymes that catabolize dopamine. Both the oxidation and, in turn, the toxic effects of MPTP can be blocked in animals before exposure to MPTP by the administration of deprenyl (Selegiline), an MAO-B inhibitor. A recent study of rodents showed that the complex I inhibitor rotenone injures nigrostriatal neurons and produces an animal model of parkinsonism.[22]

Epidemiologic studies have indicated that a number of environmental factors are associated with an increased risk of developing PD.[23,24] These include use of well water, farming, pesticides, herbicides, industrial chemicals, and rural residence. Although controversy exists regarding the role of environmental factors in the etiology of PD, it is interesting to note that herbicides and pesticides, and some agricultural products, may contain substances that inhibit mitochondrial complex I activity (see Chapter 6, *Pathogenesis*).[24]

A recent study from Harvard School of Public Health found that the incidence of PD was 70% higher in individuals exposed to pesticides than in those not exposed (adjusted relative risk 1.7; confidence interval, 1.2–2.3; $P = 0.002$.).[25] These results come from the Cancer Prevention Study II Nutrition Cohort, a longitudinal survey of US men and women initiated in 1992 by the American Cancer Society. Follow-up surveys were conducted in 1997, 1999, and 2001. Of the 143,325 individuals who returned the 2001 survey, 5.7% reported pesticide exposure. The relative risk for pesticide exposure was similar in farmers and nonfarmers.

Other exogenous toxins that affect the globus pallidus rather than the substantia nigra have been associated with the development of parkinsonism. These include trace metals, cyanide, lacquer thinner, organic solvents, carbon monoxide, and carbon disulfide.[23]

Although the epidemiologic evidence is highly suggestive, the relationship between toxin exposure and the development of PD remains poorly defined. Furthermore, no specific toxin has been identified in the brain of PD patients.

Welding has been proposed as a cause of parkinsonism. In an interesting report by Racette and others, 15 welders with parkinsonism were compared with two different control groups with idiopathic PD

(IPD).[26] In this study, however, welders were distinguished from IPD only by younger age at onset. In a more recent study, the same investigators estimated the prevalence of parkinsonism among 1,423 active male welders age 40 to 69 from Alabama who were referred for medical-legal evaluation for Parkinson's disease.[27] The prevalence ratio of parkinsonism among welders was 10.19 as compared with the age-standardized data for the general population. Thus, welding may turn out to be an environmental risk factor for IPD.

Smoking and Caffeine

■ Smoking

Many studies have shown an inverse relationship between PD and smoking, suggesting tobacco may have a symptomatic or protective effect. For example, a recent case control study of the association of environmental factors and PD found a significant inverse relationship between cigarette smoking and PD.[28] However, studies of smoking and PD have been criticized for not taking genetic factors into consideration. This criticism was addressed in a recent twin study from Sweden that investigated the associations between Parkinson's disease and smoking, as well as coffee consumption (see below), area of living, and education.[29] There was an inverse relationship between smoking and PD based on data from co-twin cases (416 same-sex twin pairs) and unrelated control subjects with and without PD.

Although the mechanisms by which smoking exerts this protective effect is not yet identified, it has been suggested that nicotine may cause increased striatal dopamine release, or that the carbon dioxide generated during cigarette smoking may have a scavenging effect on the free radicals that are produced in nigral neurons.[24]

■ Coffee and Caffeine

There have been several studies describing an inverse relationship between caffeine consumption and PD. The first large study of Japanese men showed this inverse relationship.[30] In a prospective trial with two ongoing cohorts (health professionals' follow-up study and nurses' health study), this relationship was further analyzed.[31] In men, there was a highly significant inverse relationship between coffee consumption and the risk of PD. In women, the relationship was U-shaped (ie, the lowest risk was in women consuming one to three cups per day). One explanation for this phenomenon could be that low levels of dopamine could predispose an individual to less risk for addictive behaviors, such as caffeine or nicotine use.

Summary

It is unlikely that a cause that is purely genetic or environmental will be the explanation for most cases of PD. Rather, a combination of a genetic predisposition and exposure to some as yet unidentified environmental neurotoxin may be a reasonable explanation.

REFERENCES

1. Goldman SM, Tanner C. Etiology of Parkinson's disease. In: Jankovic J, Tolosa E, eds. *Parkinson's Disease and Movement Disorders*. 3rd ed. Baltimore, Md: Lippincott-Williams and Wilkins; 1998:133-158.

2. Mikolaenko I, Pletnikova O, Kawas CH, et al. Alpha-synuclein lesions in normal aging, Parkinson disease, and Alzheimer disease: evidence from the Baltimore Longitudinal Study of Aging (BLSA). *J Neuropath Exp Neurol.* 2005;64:156-162.

3. Thal DR, Del Tredici K, Braak H. Neurodegeneration in normal drain aging and disease. *Sci Aging Knowledge Environ.* 2004;2004(23):pe26.

4. Gibb WRG, Lees AJ. Pathological clues to the cause of Parkinson's disease. In: Marsden CD, Fahn S, eds. *Movement Disorders 3*. Oxford, UK: Butterworth-Heinemann; 1994:147-165.

5. Levy G, Louis ED, Cote L, et al. Contribution of aging to the severity of different motor signs in Parkinson disease. *Arch Neurol.* 2005;62:467-472.

6. Diederich NJ, Moore CG, Leurgans SE, Chmura TA, Goetz CG. Parkinson disease with old-age onset: a comparative study with subjects with middle-age onset. *Arch Neurol.* 2003;60:529-533.

7. Tanner CM, Ottman R, Goldman SM, et al. Parkinson disease in twins: an etiologic study. *JAMA*. 1999;281:341-346.

8. Marder K, Tang MX, Mejia H, et al. Risk of Parkinson's disease among first-degree relatives: a community-based study. *Neurology*. 1996;47:155-160.

9. Lucking CB, Durr A, Bonifati V, et al. Association between early-onset Parkinson's disease and mutations in the parkin gene. French Parkinson's Disease Genetics Study Group. *N Engl J Med*. 2000;342:1560-1567.

10. Polymeropoulos MH, Lavedan C, Leroy E, et al. Mutation in the alpha-synuclein gene identified in families with Parkinson's disease. *Science.* 1997;276:2045-2047.

11. Di Fonzo A, Rohe CF, Ferreira J, et al; Italian Parkinson Genetics Network. A frequent LRRK2 gene mutation associated with autosomal dominant Parkinson's disease. *Lancet*. 2005;365:412-415.

12. Nichols WC, Pankratz N, Hernandez D, et al; Parkinson Study Group-PROGENI investigators. Genetic screening for a single common LRRK2 mutation in familial Parkinson's disease. *Lancet*. 2005;365:410-412.

13. Kachergus J, Mata IF, Hulihan M, et al. Identification of a novel LRRK2 mutation linked to autosomal dominant parkinsonism: evidence of a common founder across European populations. *Am J Hum Genet*. 2005;76:672-680.

14. Gilks WP, Abou-Sleiman PM, Gandhi S, et al. A common LRRK2 mutation in idiopathic Parkinson's disease. *Lancet*. 2005;365:415-416.

15. Deng H, Le W, Guo Y, Hunter CB, Xie W, Jankovic J. Genetic and clinical identification of Parkinson's disease patients with LRRK2 G2019S mutation. *Ann Neurol*. 2005;57: 933-934.

16. Zabetian CP, Samii A, Mosley AD, et al. A clinic-based study of the LRRK2 gene in Parkinson disease yields new mutations. *Neurology*. 2005;65:741-744.

17. Ozelius LJ, Senthil G, Saunders-Pullman R, et al. LRRK2 G2019S as a cause of Parkinson's disease in Ashkenazi Jews. *N Engl J Med*. 2006;354:424-425.

18. Hernandez D, Paisan Ruiz C, Crawley A, et al. The dardarin G 2019 S mutation is a common cause of Parkinson's disease but not other neurodegenerative diseases. *Neurosci Lett*. 2005;389:137-139.

19. Toft M, Sando SB, Melquist S, et al. LRRK2 mutations are not common in Alzheimer's disease. *Mech Ageing Dev*. 2005;126:1201-1205.

20. Kay DM, Kramer P, Higgins D, Zabetian CP, Payami H. Escaping Parkinson's disease: a neurologically healthy octogenarian with the LRRK2 G2019S mutation. *Mov Disord*. 2005;20:1077-1078.

21. Adams JR, van Netten H, Schulzer M, et al. PET in LRRK2 mutations: comparison to sporadic Parkinson's disease and evidence for presymptomatic compensation. *Brain*. 2005; 128:2777-2785.

22. Betarbet R, Sherer TB, MacKenzie G, Garcia-Osuna M, Panov AV, Greenamyre JT. Chronic system pesticide exposure reproduces features of Parkinson's disease. *Nat Neurosci*. 2000;3:1301-1306.

23. Jenner P. Current concepts on the etiology and pathogenesis of Parkinson's disease. In: 14th Annual Course. A Comprehensive Review of Movement Disorders for the Clinical Practitioner. Vol 1. Aspen, Colo; July 30-August 2, 2004:413-434.

24. Mizuno Y, Hattori N, Mochiziki H. Etiology of Parkinson's Disease. In: Watts RL, Koller WC, eds. *Movement Disorders: Neuroloogic Principles and Practice.* 2nd edition. New York, NY: The McGraw-Hill Companies; 2004:209-231.

25. Ascherio A, Chen H, Weisskopf MG, et al. Pesticide exposure and risk for Parkinson's disease. *Ann Neurol.* 2006 Jun 26; Epub ahead of print.

26. Racette BA, McGee-Minnich L, Moerlein SM, Mink JW, Videen TO, Perlmutter JS. Welding-related parkinsonism: clinical features, treatment, and pathophysiology. *Neurology.* 2001;56:8-13.

27. Racette BA, Tabbal SD, Jennings D, Good L, Perlmutter JS, Evanoff B. Prevalence of parkinsonism and relationship to exposure in a large sample of Alabama welders. *Neurology.* 2005;64:230-235.

28. Nuti A, Ceravolo R, Dell'Agnello G, et al. Environmental factors and Parkinson's disease: a case-control study in the Tuscany region of Italy. *Parkinsonism Relat Disord.* 2004; 10:481-485.

29. Wirdefeldt K, Gatz M, Pawitan Y, Pedersen NL. Risk and protective factors for Parkinson's disease: a study in Swedish twins. *Ann Neurol.* 2005;57:27-33.

30. Ross GW, Abbott RD, Petrovich H, et al. Association of coffee and caffeine intake with the risk of Parkinson disease. *JAMA.* 2000;283:2674-2679.

31. Ascherio A, Zhang SM, Hernan MA, et al. Prospective study of caffeine consumption and risk of Parkinson's disease in men and women. *Ann Neurol.* 2001;50:56-63.

4

5   Pathophysiology

The Basal Ganglia

The site of pathology responsible for the parkinsonian disorders is a group of gray matter structures within the cerebrum and ventral midbrain, the basal ganglia, generally referred to as the extrapyramidal system (**Figure 5**.1).[1] The basal ganglia include the:

- Striatum (caudate nucleus and putamen)
- Globus pallidus interna and externa
- Subthalamic nucleus
- Substantia nigra pars reticulata and pars compacta
- Intralaminar nuclei of the thalamus.

The *striatum* is composed of two parts, the caudate nucleus and putamen, which develop from the same telencephalic structure.[2] Fused together anteriorly, they serve as the input component of the basal ganglia.

The *globus pallidus* has two segments, the internal and external, the major output nucleus of the basal ganglia. Together the putamen and globus pallidus form a lens-shaped structure sometimes called the lenticular nucleus.

Because the *subthalamic nucleus* and the *substantia nigra* are closely linked to the striatum and globus pallidus, both anatomically and functionally, they are also considered to be basal ganglia. The subthalamic nucleus lies in the diencephalon, however, and the substantia nigra, in the mesencephalon.

The *substantia nigra* has two zones: a pale ventral area, the pars reticulata, which bears a cytologic resemblance to the globus pallidus, and a darkly pigmented dorsal area, the pars compacta, with nerve cell

FIGURE 5.1 — The Basal Ganglia

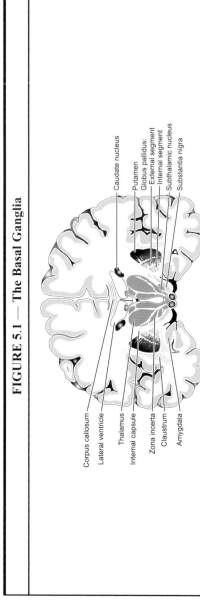

Seen here in relation to their surrounding structures, the basal ganglia include the caudate nucleus and putamen (striatum), the globus pallidus (external and internal segments), the subthalamic nucleus, and the substantia nigra (pars compacta and pars reticulata), and the intralaminar nuclei of the thalamus.

Adapted from: Kandel ER, et al, eds. *Principles of Neural Science*. 4th ed. New York, NY: The McGraw Hill Companies; 2000:853-867.

bodies that contain neuromelanin, a polymer of dopamine or its metabolites (**Figure 5.2**).[3] The neurons of the pars compacta use dopamine as a transmitter, but the function of the pigment is uncertain.

FIGURE 5.2 — The Normal Substantia Nigra

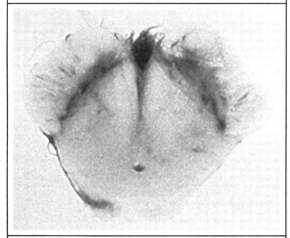

The normal substantia nigra with its melanin-pigmented pars compacta.

Intrathalamic nuclei provide the entrance and exit pathways from the cerebral cortex to the basal ganglia and back.

The basal ganglia have separate input and output components, as well as a series of internuclear connections, mediated by specific neurotransmitters (**Figure 5.3**).[4]

Major sources of afferent pathways arising from extrinsic neuronal groups include:

- Neocortex to the striatum, mediated by the neurotransmitter glutamate (other, as yet unidentified neurotransmitters may also be involved)
- Thalamic nonspecific nuclei to the striatum, using glutamate[4]

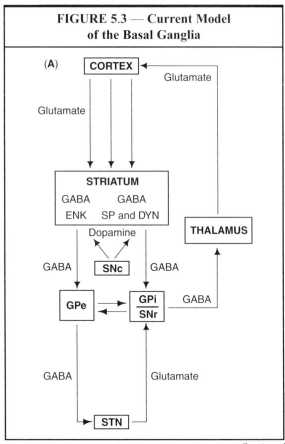

FIGURE 5.3 — Current Model of the Basal Ganglia

Continued

- Locus ceruleus to the substantia nigra, via norepinephrine
- Dorsal raphé, nucleus and raphé, nucleus to striatum and substantia nigra, respectively, using serotonin.

The major efferent pathways from the basal ganglia to the extrinsic neuronal groups include:

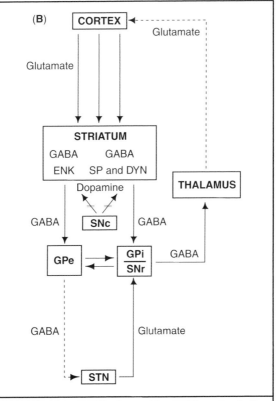

(B)

Abbreviations: DYN, dynorphin; ENK, enkephalin; GABA, gamma-aminobutyric acid; GPe, globus pallidus externa; GPi, globus pallidus interna; SNc, substantia nigra pars compacta; SNr, substantia nigra pars reticulata; SP, substance P; STN, subthalamic nucleus.

The diagrams illustrate the functional organization of the basal ganglia in (A) normal conditions and (B) Parkinson's disease.

Parent A, et al. *Trends Neurosci.* 2000;23(10 suppl):S21.

- Substantia nigra pars reticulata (SNr) and globus pallidus interna (GPi) to thalamic nuclei using gamma-aminobutyric acid (GABA)
- Thalamic nuclei to cortex, using glutamate.[4]

The nuclear groups of the basal ganglia are closely interconnected. The putamen and substantia nigra have prominent reciprocal connections mediated by specific inhibitory or excitatory neurotransmitters[3,4]:

- From striatum to SNr and GPi, mediated by the inhibitory neurotransmitter GABA and substance P (SP)
- From substantia nigra pars compacta (SNc) to striatum, mediated by dopamine (DA).

The other connections are made by two functional dopaminergic systems that are in relative balance. An indirect pathway, through which DA normally inhibits transmission, projects[3,4]:

- From striatum to globus pallidus externa (GPe), mediated by GABA and enkephalin
- From GPe to subthalamic nucleus (STN), using GABA
- From STN to SNr and GPi, using glutamate
- From SNr and GPi to ventrolateral nucleus of the thalamus, using GABA
- From thalamus to cortex, using glutamate.[4]

A direct pathway, with transmission facilitated by DA, projects from:

- Striatum to GPi, mediated by GABA, SP, and dynorphin
- GPi to ventralis lateralis (VL) of thalamus
- Thalamus to cortex.

The striatum is driven by excitatory input from all major sensory and motor regions of the cerebral cortex, as well as the thalamic nuclei, via the excitatory thalamostriatal connection.[4] Both of these excitatory pathways use glutamate as their transmitter, with its principal targets being the inotropic AMPA (α-amino-3-hydroxy-5-methylisoxazole-4-propionic acid)- and NMDA (N-methyl-D-aspartate)-type glutamate receptors.

Direct striatal output via GABAergic, hence inhibitory, striatonigral and striatopallidal neurons, although normally electrically quiescent, can be driven by acetylcholine and glutamate. If glutamate or acetylcholine stimulates the direct striatal output pathway, it reduces inhibitory tone in nigrothalamic fibers, increases excitation in the feedback loop to the premotor cortex, and thereby permits movement.

On the other hand, when these same transmitters act on the indirect pathway, they bring about a sequence of events that ultimately sends exactly the opposite signals back to the cortex, thus prohibiting movement. Therefore, the net balance between glutamate's physiologic stimulant activity on the excitatory and inhibitory executive pathways of the striatum determines whether the basal ganglia issue instructions for motor acts to proceed or not.

At the striatal level, dopamine appears to facilitate transmission along the direct pathway and inhibit transmission along the indirect pathway using D_1 and D_2 receptors, respectively.[4,5] Imbalance in the activity of the direct and indirect pathway and the resultant alterations in circuitry are thought to account for the features of Parkinson's disease and other basal ganglia disorders (eg, the hyperkinetic movement disorder Huntington's disease).

Thus the circuitry's distinct neurotransmitter anatomy permits modulation of the motor cortex's output, apparently to aid in the generation of commands concerned with controlling proximal muscle groups during movements.[1] It monitors ongoing movement in order to prepare the motor system for the next movement in a sequence. When a particular behavior is selected, the appropriate neurons can be excited, inhibited, and disinhibited to facilitate and maintain motor programs, with emphasis on suppression of unwanted movements. The basal ganglia are instrumental in unconscious "automatic" reflexes that underlie such activities as eating, adjustment of posture, and defensive reactions.

Dopamine

Synthesized in the brain's dopaminergic neurons and other neurons from the amino acid L-tyrosine via the intermediate compound, L-3,4-dihydroxyphenylalanine (levodopa), dopamine is then concentrated in the neurons' storage vesicles. Under physiologic conditions, dopamine is released by a calcium-dependent mechanism into the synaptic cleft, where it may bind to either[5]:

- Postsynaptic receptors on target cells
- Autoreceptors, specific cell-surface receptors on the same neuron.

Dopamine is inactivated primarily by the reuptake process, after which it may be sequestered again in storage vesicles for release. It is also inactivated enzymatically by the action of both monoamine oxidase type B (MAO-B), an enzyme associated with mitochondria and present in two forms, A and B, and by catechol-0-methyltransferase (COMT), an enzyme localized primarily in the brain's glial cells. The principal metabolite of dopamine is homovanillic acid (HVA).

Physiologically, the striatonigral and striatal-GPe pathways appear to be excited by the action of dopamine, whereas the striatal-GPi pathway is inhibited by it. Dopamine's capacity to reverse the bradykinesia, rigidity, and tremor caused by dopamine depletion seems to require action at both receptor types.

■ Dopamine Receptors

At least six different forms of the dopamine receptor are now known, categorized under two main types D_1-like and D_2-like.[5] The D_1 type, which is generally stimulatory, is divided into two subtypes:

- D_1
- D_5.

The D_2, inhibitory, type includes:

- D_{2short}
- D_{2long}
- D_3
- D_4.

The pharmacological profile and regional distribution in brain of each subtype is different, with the exception of D_{2short} and D_{2long}, which appear to be identical in these respects. D_1 and D_2 receptors are present in medium spiny neurons throughout the striatum, whereas D_3 receptors are confined to the limbic-related ventral striatum.

Although it is now established that the stimulatory and inhibitory pathways act synergistically in the expression of certain behaviors, the neuroanatomical basis for the interaction is not clear. It appears, however, that striatal D_1-like receptors are expressed predominantly by striatonigral and striatopallidal neurons that are GABAergic and also express SP.[5]

In contrast, D_2-like receptors seem to be expressed primarily by substantia nigra dopaminergic neurons (autoreceptors), cholinergic interneurons in the striatum, and striatopallidal neurons projecting to the GPe, which are GABAergic and coexpress enkephalin.

■ Dopamine's Role in Parkinson's Disease

The foremost pathological characteristic of Parkinson's disease (PD) is the death of pigmented dopamine neurons in the SNc. Overt parkinsonism does not present until approximately 80% of striatal dopamine loss has occurred, however.[6] The remaining nigrostriatal neurons mount a compensatory response to severe losses by increasing the rate of dopamine synthesis and release.

Another compensatory mechanism is a reduction in the rate of dopamine inactivation. As the number of dopamine nerve terminals in the striatum decreases, so does the density of dopamine uptake sites, which comprise the primary mechanism for regulating the synaptic concentration of dopamine.[5] Thus, dopamine in the extracellular fluid can diffuse further and persist for a longer period than normal, providing the potential for it to interact with more distant postsynaptic dopamine receptors than normally.

Eventual decompensation results in an imbalance in the equilibrium between the direct and indirect striatal output pathways, however.[4] In the absence of dopamine, the driving of striatopallidal GABAergic neurons by glutamate goes unchecked. The loss of D_2 inhibitory control, both pre- and postsynaptically in the striatum, leads to a pronounced increase in basal ganglia inhibitory output from the indirect pathway, giving rise to the classical symptoms of rigidity and akinesia.

The Parkinson Lesion

The primary lesion of PD is degeneration of the neuromelanin-containing neurons in the brain stem, particularly those in the pars compacta of the substantia nigra, which becomes visibly pale to the naked eye (**Figure 5.4**).[7] Microscopically, the pigmented nuclei show a marked depletion of cells and replacement gliosis.

The surviving neurons are likely to contain Lewy bodies, the pathologic hallmark of PD (**Figure 5.5**).[7] These eosinophilic inclusion bodies found within the cytoplasm of neurons in the cerebral cortex and lim-

FIGURE 5.4 — The Parkinson Lesion

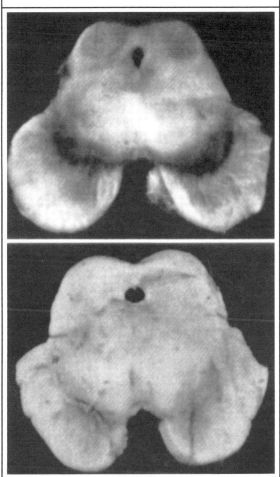

(Top) Normally pigmented substantia nigra. *(Bottom)* Substantia nigra of a patient with Parkinson's Disease.

Watts RL, Koller WC, eds. *Movement Disorders: Neurologic Principles and Practice*. 2nd ed. New York, NY: The McGraw-Hill Companies; 2004:145.

5

FIGURE 5.5 — The Lewy Body

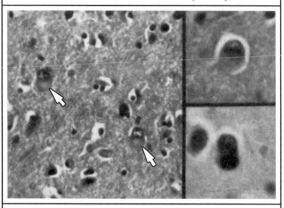

Cortical Lewy bodies *(arrows)* in two neurons *(left,* hematoxylin-eosin stain); single cortical Lewy body at higher magnification *(upper right,* hematoxylin-eosin stain); single cortical Lewy body *(lower right,* α-synuclein immunohistochemistry).

Watts RL, Koller WC, eds. *Movement Disorders: Neurologic Principles and Practice*. 2nd ed. New York, NY: The McGraw-Hill Companies; 2004:146.

bic system. By electron microscopy, the predominant structural component of the Lewy body is seen to be filamentous material arranged in circular and linear profiles, sometimes radiating from an electron-dense core. A weakly staining second inclusion, called a pale body, is also found frequently but not invariably. It consists of a very sparse accumulation of neurofilament interspersed with vacuoles and granular bodies. The cause of this excessive accumulation of filamentous material within surviving neurons is unknown.

It is now known that the vesicle-associated protein, α-synuclein, is the key constituent of the Lewy body.[9] Although other filamentous proteins are associated with Lewy bodies, α-synuclein is considered to play a central role in the pathogenesis of PD.[8]

Although Lewy bodies are present in PD, they are also found in a few other rare neurodegenerative diseases. The most recently recognized of these, dementia with Lewy bodies (DLB), is differentiated from PD by widespread cortical and subcortical Lewy body formation and the invariable development of dementia (see Chapter 7, *Diagnosis*). The cortical Lewy bodies are more difficult to detect. They are poorly defined areas of cytoplasmic condensation. Both classical and cortical Lewy bodies share immunoreactivity to neurofilament, ubiquitin, and α-synuclein.[8]

5

REFERENCES

1. Kandel ER, Schwartz JH, Jessell TM, eds. *Principles of Neural Science*. 4th ed. New York, NY: The McGraw-Hill Companies; 2000:853-867.

2. Nolte J, ed. *The Human Brain: An Introduction to Its Functional Anatomy*. 2nd ed. St. Louis, Mo: The CV Mosby Company; 1988.

3. Wooten GF. Neurochemistry and neuropharmacology of Parkinson's disease. In: Watts RL, Koller WC, eds. *Movement Disorders: Neurologic Principles and Practice*. 2nd ed. New York, NY: The McGraw-Hill Companies; 1997:153-160.

4. Parent A, Sato F, Wu Y, Gauthier J, Levesque M, Parent M. Organization of the basal ganglia: the importance of axonal collateralization. *Trends Neurosci*. 2000;23(10 suppl):S20-S27.

5. Micheli F, Cersosimo MG, Wooten GF. Neurochemistry and Neuropharmacology of Parkinson's disease. In: Watts RL, Koller WC, eds. *Movement Disorders: Neurologic Principles and Practice*. 2nd ed. New York, NY: The McGraw-Hill Companies; 2004:197-207.

6. Jankovic J, Marsden CD. Therapeutic strategies in Parkinson's disease. In: Jankovic J, Tolosa E, eds. *Parkinson's Disease and Movement Disorders*. Baltimore, Md: Urban and Schwarzenberg; 1988:95-119.

7. Gearing M, Mirra SS. Neuropathology of movement disorders: an overview. In: Watts RL, Koller WC, eds. *Movement Disorders: Neurologic Principles and Practice*. 2nd ed. New York, NY: The McGraw-Hill Companies; 2004:143-158.

8. Wainer BH, Stover NP. Parkinson's disease: neuropathology. In: Watts RL, Koller WC, eds. *Movement Disorders: Neurologic Principles and Practice*. 2nd ed. New York, NY: The McGraw-Hill Companies; 2004:327-336.

6 Pathogenesis

Complex molecular mechanisms underlying the pathogenesis of Parkinson's disease (PD) are gradually being elucidated. Several factors and processes seem to be involved in the pathogenesis of PD including:[1-7]

- Oxidative stress
- Ubiquitin-proteasome system (UPS) dysfunction
- Mitochondrial dysfunction
- Excitotoxicity
- Inflammation.

Detailed reviews of these factors are beyond the scope of this chapter. However, brief overviews follow.

Oxidative Stress

Oxidative damage to high molecular weight substances, such as proteins, lipids, and nucleic acids, is found in the substantia nigra (SN) of patients with PD.[3,4] Postmortem studies in patients who died with PD indicate that a variety of biomolecules have undergone oxidative damage. Oxidative stress may also damage nuclear and mitochondrial DNA.

Oxidative stress occurs when the equilibrium is disturbed between antioxidant defense mechanisms and factors that promote free radical formation.[8] Aerobic cells use molecular oxygen as the terminal electron acceptor in oxidative phosphorylation. Therefore, these cells must be capable of dealing with the side effects of oxygen and its reactive derivatives that are, in the following order of reduction from oxygen:

- Superoxide anion radicals
- Hydrogen peroxide
- Hydroxy radicals.

Under physiologic conditions, superoxide is readily reduced to hydrogen peroxide, oxygen, and water by enzymes, such as superoxide dismutase, catalase, and glutathione peroxidase, or by interaction with transitional metals. Peroxide is relatively unreactive toward organic compounds. However, its interaction with transitional metals (copper, iron) generates the more reactive hydroxyl radical, which can induce apoptosis (see below) in rat cortical neurons. Hydroxyl radicals are highly toxic and can combine with or abstract moieties from practically any biological molecule, including DNA, protein, and lipid membranes.

The brain appears to be particularly vulnerable to oxidative stress. Neuronal membranes contain a high proportion of radical-susceptible polyunsaturated fatty acids. Moreover, the brain's antioxidant defenses are weak. With low levels of glutathione (GSH), almost no catalase, and comparatively low concentrations of both GSH peroxidase and vitamin E, the relatively high oxygen consumption of the brain makes it susceptible to physiologic disequilibrium with resultant oxidative stress.

The SN is rich in dopamine, which can undergo both monoamine oxidase (MAO)-mediated and auto-oxidation to neuromelanin, hydrogen peroxide, and free radicals. These agents overwhelm the normally protective effects of vitamin E (alpha tocopherol) and GSH peroxidase, which remove hydrogen peroxides and lipid peroxide.[9]

Oxidative stress most likely contributes to the cascade of events that leads to dopaminergic cell degeneration in PD. However, oxidative stress is also intimately linked to other components of the degenerative process, such as mitochondrial dysfunction, excitotoxicity, and inflammation (see discussions below).[10-12]

Ubiquitin-Proteasome System Dysfunction

The UPS is a multicomponent pathway that identifies abnormal proteins and tags them for degradation by the 26/20S proteasome.[13,14] Proteins that inhibit proteasomal function have also recently been identified. These agents seem to regulate proteasomal activity and prevent excessive and undesired destruction of native proteins. In addition to clearing unwanted proteins, the UPS helps regulate important transcriptional and transmitter proteins within the cell.

Impairment in the capacity of the UPS to clear aberrant, misfolded, and potentially cytotoxic proteins may be an important factor in the pathogenesis of the various forms of PD.[6,7,14-16]

■ The UPS and Parkinson's Disease

The hallmarks of PD are the preferential degeneration of dopaminergic neurons in the substantia nigra pars compacta (SNpc) and the accumulation of poorly degraded proteins in intracytoplasmic inclusions (Lewy bodies). Recently, several converging lines of evidence have demonstrated a link between the inhibition of UPS function, dopaminergic neuronal degeneration, and the accumulation of abnormal proteins.

McNaught and colleagues showed that inhibition of the UPS in fetal rat ventral mesencephalic cultures caused degeneration of dopaminergic neurons with accumulation of proteinaceous inclusions consisting of α-synuclein and ubiquitin.[15] A subsequent study by the same investigators found a synergistic effect on dopaminergic cell death when inhibition of proteasomal activity was combined with conditions that promote protein damage and misfolding, such as oxidative stress and heat shock.[17]

A recent *in vivo* study also revealed a direct relationship between inhibition of proteasomal function, accumulation of α-synuclein inclusions, and degeneration of nigrostriatal dopaminergic neurons in the SNpc.[18] After unilateral intrastriatal injection of the selective proteasome inhibitor lactacystin, dopaminergic neurons in the ipsilateral SNpc progressively degenerated and contained α-synuclein–immunopositive intracytoplasmic inclusions. When high concentrations of lactacystin were injected, the striatum was simultaneously involved, and α-synuclein extracytoplasmic inclusions appeared extensively throughout the SN. In addition, increased levels of heme oxygenase-1, a marker of oxidative stress, were associated with degeneration of the dopaminergic neurons.

An animal model was created in rats that received systemic injections of proteosome inhibitors over a 2-week period.[19] After a latency of 1 to 2 weeks, the animals developed parkinsonism with bradykinesia, rigidity, tremor, and abnormal posture; this improved with apomorphine treatment. Striatal dopamine depletion, dopaminergic cell death, and intracytoplasmic α-synuclein and ubiquitin-containing inclusions resembling Lewy bodies were noted at autopsy.

A decline in UPS activity due to environmental or genetic reasons (see later) may explain the irreversible loss of dopamine neurons that characterize PD.[6]

Mitochondrial Injury and Dysfunction

Postmortem brain material from PD patients has shown a decrease in complex I activity in the substantia nigra compacta (SNc).[20,21] This defect was not found in other brain areas in PD patients, nor was it seen elsewhere in brains of patients with multiple system atrophy (MSA) and other neurodegenerative disorders in which there is extensive degeneration of nigrostriatal neurons. A similar defect in complex I has been reported in platelets, fibroblasts, and muscle of patients with PD, although these findings are less consistent.[22,23]

The first clue to understanding mitochondrial dysfunction in PD came with the elucidation of the mechanism of action of methylphenyltetrahydropyridine (MPTP).[24] After conversion by monoamine oxidase type B (MAO-B), the neurotoxin's product, methylphenylpyridinium ion (MPP$^+$), is actively taken up into dopaminergic neurons and concentrated in mitochondria. Here, it specifically inhibits complex I (NADH CoQ1 reductase), the first enzyme of the respiratory chain. The resulting decrease in ATP synthesis is thought to account for the death of the dopamine-containing neurons.

Analysis of respiratory chain activity in the Parkinson brain has shown a 37% decrease in complex I activity, with normal activity of complexes II to IV. This selective deficiency in complex I activity seems to be confined to the SN, particularly the pars compacta.[25] However, not all PD patients express a defect in complex I, and it is not yet known to what degree this reduction in complex I activity found in some patients can induce a bioenergetic deficit.[3] It is felt that mitochondrial dysfunction can lead to a number of deleterious consequences, including impaired calcium buffering, generation of free radicals, and secondary excitotoxicity.[26,27]

Recent evidence has implicated mitochondria in apoptotic cell death.[28] Apoptosis is associated with a decrease in mitochondrial membrane potential and opening of a mitochondrial permeability transition pore. The release of small proteins then signals the initiation of apoptosis. The decrease in complex I activity could impair proton pumping and make nigral cells vulnerable to apoptosis.

Regardless of the initial insult, a cascade of events involving both oxygen radicals and mitochondrial metabolism is likely to contribute to cell injury.

Excitotoxicity

Excitotoxicity occurring in response to a rise in glutamate or glutaminergic transmission has been implicated in the pathogenesis of PD and other neurodegenerative diseases.[26,29,30] In the normal brain, concentration of excitatory amino acids (EAAs) is maintained within the synaptic cleft at subtoxic levels, with rapid uptake and inactivation by both neurons and glia. However, a defect in mitochondrial function, specifically diminished activity of complex I of the electron transport chain, presumably causes a bioenergetic defect in the dopamine neurons of the substantia nigra, reducing their capacity to maintain a normal membrane potential. Thus voltage-dependent N-methyl-D-aspartate (NMDA) ion channels are more easily activated, leading to slow excitotoxic neuronal death.

Inflammation

The immunohistochemical demonstration of activated microglia and activated complement components in affected brain regions in PD suggests that chronic inflammation may play a role in the pathogenesis of PD.[5] Elevated levels of inflammatory cytokines and tumor necrosis factor-α (TNF-α) were found in the PD brain in one study.[3] MPTP studies show that inflammation can persist for many years after the initial stimulus has disappeared.[31]

Inflammation can also generate, or contribute to, oxidative stress. One mechanism is via the release of superoxide ions generated and released by the respiratory burst system of activated microglia as part of their purposeful attack system.[31] Evidence of free-radical attack in the SN in PD includes the presence of proteins modified by glycation, oxidized and nitrated low molecular weight compounds, and peroxidated lipids.[5]

Zhang and coworkers demonstrated that the addition of human extracellular aggregated α-synuclein resulted in activation of microglia.[32] This, in turn, enhanced aggregated α-synuclein–mediated neurodegeneration. Furthermore, microglial activation and phagocytosis of aggregated α-synuclein led to activation of NADPH oxidase and production of reactive oxygen species (ROS). These investigators suggested that nigral neuronal damage may release aggregated α-synuclein into the SN. Subsequent microglial activation and production of proinflammatory mediators could lead to persistent and progressive nigral degeneration in PD.

These, and other lines of evidence, support the hypothesis that chronic inflammation may play an important although, perhaps, a secondary role in the pathogenesis of PD.

Apoptosis

The mode of neuron death in degenerative diseases is now thought to probably occur via apoptosis, a morphologically unique process of cell death that is distinct from necrosis. Necrotic death results from severe and sudden thermal, physical, or chemical trauma and characterized by early mitochondrial and cellular swelling, with ensuing cytoskeletal disruption and ruptured plasma membrane and organelles. The nuclear structure ultimately becomes disrupted as well.

Apoptosis is a sequential process that starts with condensation of chromatin and loss of cell volume.[33] The plasma membrane becomes ruffled and blebbed. Nucleus and cytoplasm are partitioned into membrane-bound apoptotic bodies that are shed from the dying cells. In the last stages, most cells display a characteristic degradation of nuclear DNA into multimers of 180 bp (DNA laddering). Throughout the process, the mitochondria remain morphologically normal. Neighboring cells subsequently phagocytize the dying cell.

Neurons die by apoptosis during development of the brain. Apoptosis can be induced by removal of trophic factors from primary cultures of neurons.[8] The apoptotic pathway is regulated by the levels of certain apoptosis-related genes.

The involvement of apoptosis in neurodegenerative diseases was shown by exposure of cultured neurons to a range of conditions characteristic of those disorders, all of which induce cell death by apoptosis:

- GSH depletion
- Chronic inhibition of superoxide dismutase
- β-Amyloid fragments
- Dopamine
- Ischemia.

Summary

There are multiple, interrelated factors and biomolecular processes that contribute to the pathogenesis of PD. Oxidative stress, UPS and mitochondrial dysfunction, excitotoxicity, and inflammation may play major roles in the progressive degeneration of dopaminergic neurons in PD. Genetic and environmental influences (see Chapter 4, *Etiology*) may further impact these processes.

REFERENCES

1. Bossy-Wetzel E, Schwarzenbacher R, Lipton SA. Molecular pathways to neurodegeneration. *Nat Med.* 2004;10(suppl): S2-S9.

2. Moore DJ, West AB, Dawson VL, et al. Molecular pathophysiology of Parkinson's disease. *Annu Rev Neurosci.* 2005; January 25 [Epub ahead of print].

3. Jenner P. Current concepts on the etiology and pathogenesis of Parkinson's disease. In: 14th Annual Course. A Comprehensive Review of Movement Disorders for the Clinical Practitioner. Vol 1. Aspen, Colo; July 30-August 2, 2004:413-434.

4. Mizuno Y, Hattori N, Mochizuki H. Etiology of Parkinson's disease. In: Watts RL, Koller WC, eds, *Movement Disorders: Neurologic Principles and Practice.* 2nd ed. New York, NY: The McGraw-Hill Companies; 2004:209-231.

5. McGeer PL, McGeer EG. Inflammation and neurodegeneration in Parkinson's disease. *Parkinsonism Relat Disord.* 2004;10(suppl 1):S3-S7.

6. Eriksen JL, Wszolek A, Petrucelli L. Molecular pathogenesis of Parkinson disease. *Arch Neurol.* 2005;62:353-357.

7. Petrucelli L, Dawson TM. Mechanism of neurodegenerative disease: role of the ubiquitin proteosome system. *Ann Med.* 2004;36:315-320.

8. Gorman AM, McGowan A, O'Neill C, Cotter T. Oxidative stress and apoptosis in neurodegeneration. *J Neurol Sci.* 1996;139(suppl):45-52.

9. Cohen G. The brain on fire? *Ann Neurol.* 1994;36:333-334.

10. Jenner P. Oxidative stress in Parkinson's disease. *Ann Neurol.* 2003;53(suppl 3):S26-S36.

11. Beal MF. Mitochondria, oxidative damage, and inflammation in Parkinson's disease. *Ann N Y Acad Sci.* 2003;991: 120-131.

12. Emerit J, Edeas M, Bricaire F. Neurodegenerative disease and oxidative stress. *Biomed Pharmacother.* 2004;58:39-46.

13. Sherman MY, Goldberg AL. Cellular defenses against unfolded proteins: a cell biologist thinks about neurodegenerative diseases. *Neuron.* 2001;29:15-32.

14. McNaught KS, Olanow CW, Halliwell B, Isacson O, Jenner P. Failure of the ubiquitin-proteasome system in Parkinson's disease. *Nat Rev Neurosci.* 2001;2:589-594.

15. McNaught KS, Mytilineou C, Jnobaptiste R, et al. Impairment of the ubiquitin-proteasome system causes dopaminergic cell death and inclusion body formation in ventral mesencephalic cultures. *J Neurochem.* 2002;81:301-306.

16. Ross CA, Pickart CM. The ubiquitin-proteasome pathway in Parkinson's disease and other neurodegenerative diseases. *Trends Cell Biol.* 2004;14:703-711.

17. Mytilineou C, McNaught KS, Shashidharan P, et al. Inhibition of proteasome activity sensitizes dopamine neurons to protein alterations and oxidative stress. *J Neural Transm.* 2004;111:1237-1251.

18. Miwa H, Kubo R, Suzuki A, Nishi K, Kondo T. Retrograde dopaminergic neuron degeneration following intrastriatal proteasome inhibition. *Neurosci Lett.* 2005;380:93-98.

19. McNaught KS, Perl DP, Brownell AL, Olanow CW. Systemic exposure to proteasome inhibitors causes a progressive model of Parkinson's disease. *Ann Neurol.* 2004;56:149-162.

20. Schapira AHV, Cooper JM, Dexter D, Clark JB, Jenner P, Marsden CD. Mitochondrial complex I deficiency in Parkinson's disease. *J Neurochem.* 1990;54:823-827.

21. Mizuno Y, Ohta S, Tanaka M, et al. Deficiencies in complex I subunits of the respiratory chain in Parkinson's disease. *Biochem Biophys Res Commun.* 1989;163:1450-1455.

22. Schapira AH. Evidence for mitochondrial dysfunction in Parkinson's disease: a critical appraisal. *Mov Disord.* 1994;9:125-138.

23. DiMauro S. Mitochondrial involvement in Parkinson's disease: the controversy continues. *Neurology.* 1993;43:2170-2172.

24. Krige D, Carroll MT, Cooper JM, Marsden CD, Shapira AH. Platelet mitochondrial function in Parkinson's disease. The Royal Kings and Queens Parkinson's Disease Research Group. *Ann Neurol.* 1992;32:782-788.

25. Schapira AH, Gu M, Taanman JW, et al. Mitochondria in the etiology and pathogenesis of Parkinson's disease. *Ann Neurol.* 1998;44(3 suppl 1):S89-S98.

26. Beal MF. Excitotoxicity and nitric acid in Parkinson's disease pathogenesis. *Ann Neurol.* 1998;44(3 suppl 1):S110-S114.

27. Byrne E. Does mitochondrial respiratory chain dysfunction have a role in common neurodegenerative disorders? *J Clin Neurosci.* 2002;9:497-501.

28. Tatton WG, Olanow CW. Apoptosis in neurodegenerative disease: the role of the mitochondria. *Biochem Biophys Acta.* 1999;1410:195-213.

29. Choi D. Glutamate neurotoxicity and diseases of the nervous system. *Neuron.* 1988;1:623-634.

30. Beal MF. Role of excitotoxicity in human neurological disease. *Curr Opin Neurobiol.* 1992;2:657-662.

31. McGeer PL, McGeer EG. Inflammation and the degenerative diseases of aging. *Ann N Y Acad Sci.* 2004;1035:104-116.

32. Zhang W, Wang T, Pei Z, et al. Aggregated alpha-synuclein activates microglia: a process leading to disease progression in Parkinson's disease. *FASEB J.* 2005;19:533-542.

33. Lee WMF, Dang CV. Control of cell growth, differentiation, and death. In: Hoffman R, Benz EJ Jr, et al, eds. *Hematology: Basic Principles and Practice.* 2nd ed. New York, NY: Churchill Livingstone; 1995:81.

7   Diagnosis

The cardinal signs and symptoms of Parkinson's disease (PD), when present in their entirety, impart the well-known, unmistakable clinical picture of resting tremor, rigidity, akinesia, and impairment of postural reflexes. It evolves slowly, however, with early symptoms so mild as to escape notice by either patients or those close to them. This prediagnostic period may last for years.

Initial presentation is seldom the full-blown disease. Individual physical findings are not specific to the disease; each may herald one or more long-latency parkinsonian syndromes.[1] In many cases, therefore, PD is a diagnosis of exclusion rather than a straightforward presentation of a specific deficit profile. When not all of the signs are evident, there is no alternative but to reexamine the patient at several-month intervals until it is clear that PD is present or the signature of another degenerative process becomes evident (**Table 7.1**).[1]

Clinical Diagnosis

The main difficulty in the clinical diagnosis of PD is to distinguish the disease from the parkinsonian syndromes as well as other conditions that resemble specific features of either.[1-3]

Gelb and colleagues divided the clinical features of PD into two groups according to their diagnostic utility:

- Group A included features characteristic of PD
- Group B are features suggestive of alternate diagnoses (**Table 7.2**).[2]

TABLE 7.1 — Motor and Nonmotor Manifestations of Parkinson's Disease

Cardinal Manifestations
- Rest tremor
- Rigidity
- Akinesia/bradykinesia
- Postural instability

Secondary Manifestations
- Cognitive/neuropsychiatric
- Anxiety
- Bradyphrenia
- Dementia
- Depression
- Sleep disorders

Cardinal Nerve/Facial
- Blurred vision (impaired upgaze, blepharospasm)
- Dysarthria
- Dysphagia
- Glabellar reflex (Myerson's sign)
- Olfactory dysfunction
- Sialorrhea (drooling)

Musculoskeletal
- Compression neuropathies
- Dystonia
- Hand and foot deformities
- Kyphoscoliosis
- Peripheral edema

Autonomic
- Constipation
- Orthostatic hypotension/lightheadedness
- Increased sweating
- Sexual dysfunction (impotence, loss of libido)
- Urinary dysfunction (frequency, hesitancy, urgency)

Continued

Sensory
- Cramps
- Olfactory dysfunction
- Pain
- Paresthesias
- Restless legs syndrome

Skin
- Seborrhea

Adapted from: Paulson HL, Stern MB. *Movement Disorders: Neurologic Principles and Practice*. 2nd ed. New York, NY: The McGraw-Hill Companies; 2004:233-245.

TABLE 7.2 — Grouping of Clinical Features According to Diagnostic Utility

7

Group A Features: Characteristic of Parkinson's Disease
- Resting tremor
- Bradykinesia
- Rigidity
- Asymmetric onset

Group B Features: Suggestive of Alternative Diagnoses
- Features unusual early in the clinical course
  – Prominent postural instability in the first 3 years after symptom onset
  – Freezing phenomena in the first 3 years
  – Hallucinations unrelated to medications in the first 3 years
  – Dementia preceding motor symptoms or in the first year
- Supranuclear gaze palsy (other than restriction of upward gaze) or slowing of vertical saccades
- Severe, symptomatic dysautonomia unrelated to medications
- Documentation of a condition known to produce parkinsonism and plausibly connected to the patient's symptoms (such as suitably located focal brain lesions or neuroleptic use within the past 6 months)

Adapted from: Gelb DJ, et al. *Arch Neurol* 1999;56:33-39.

Based on combinations of Group A and Group B clinical features, proposed diagnostic criteria for Parkinson's disease were formulated that provide three levels of diagnostic confidence: Definite, Probable, and Possible (**Table 7.3**).[2] However, they noted while diagnoses of Possible and Probable PD are based on clinical criteria, the diagnosis of Definite PD requires neuropathologic confirmation.

TABLE 7.3 — Proposed Diagnostic Criteria for Parkinson's Disease

POSSIBLE Diagnosis of Parkinson's Disease
At least 2 of the 4 Group A features are present; at least 1 of them is tremor or bradykinesia

and

Either: None of the Group B features is present
Or: Symptoms have been present for <3 years, and none of the Group B features is present to date.

and

Either: Substantial and sustained response to levodopa or a dopamine agonist has been documented
Or: Patient has not had an adequate trial of levodopa or dopamine agonist

PROBABLE Diagnosis of Parkinson's Disease
At least 3 of the 4 Group A features are present

and

None of the Group B features is present (symptom duration of at least 3 years duration is necessary to meet this requirement)

and

Substantial and sustained response to levodopa or a dopamine agonist has been documented

DEFINITE Diagnosis of Parkinson's Disease
All criteria of POSSIBLE Parkinson's disease are met

and

Histopathologic confirmation of the diagnosis is obtained at autopsy

Adapted from: Gelb DJ, et al. *Arch Neurol* 1999;56:33-39.

An alternate approach to clinical differentiation of PD and atypical parkinsonian disorders was recently proposed by Christine and associates (**Figure** 7.1).[3] This approach focuses on selected clinical features such as slow versus rapid development of signs and symptoms, key signs and symptoms, and response to levodopa or a dopamine agonist.

■ **Essential Tremor**

Rest tremor is the best known and most readily identifiable early sign of PD and it is the first motor manifestation in about 75% of patients.[1,4] However, it can sometimes be difficult to differentiate it from other relatively common types of tremor, such as essential tremor.

Essential tremor (**Figure** 7.2) is a heredofamilial action tremor that usually begins in early adult life and typically is progressive and potentially disabling. Essential tremor is distinguished from that of PD by:[4,5]

- Its low amplitude and higher frequency
- A tendency to become manifest during volitional movement and to disappear when the limb is in repose
- Lack of associated slowness of movement, flexed postures, etc.

Some slower, alternating forms of essential tremor are difficult to distinguish from parkinsonian tremor. Comparative characteristics of the two are listed in **Table** 7.4.

The majority of patients with hypokinetic disorders referred to specialized movement disorder clinics are diagnosed clinically as having PD (**Table** 7.5).[6] The second most common group, including progressive supranuclear palsy (PSP), multiple system atrophy (MSA), corticobasal degeneration (CBD), and dementia with Lewy bodies (DLB), have been categorized clinically as "parkinsonism plus disorders." Others,

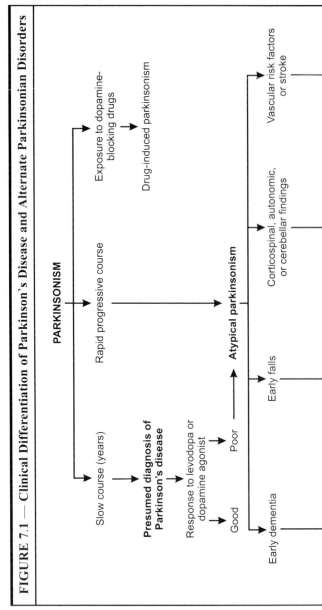

FIGURE 7.1 — Clinical Differentiation of Parkinson's Disease and Alternate Parkinsonian Disorders

PARKINSONISM

Slow course (years) → **Presumed diagnosis of Parkinson's disease** → Response to levodopa or dopamine agonist

Good → Early dementia

Poor → **Atypical parkinsonism**

Rapid progressive course → **Atypical parkinsonism**

Exposure to dopamine-blocking drugs → Drug-induced parkinsonism

Early falls

Corticospinal, autonomic, or cerebellar findings

Vascular risk factors or stroke

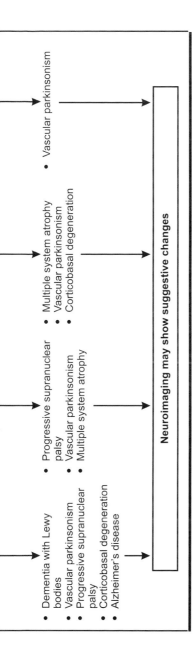

- Dementia with Lewy bodies
- Vascular parkinsonism
- Progressive supranuclear palsy
- Corticobasal degeneration
- Alzheimer's disease

- Progressive supranuclear palsy
- Vascular parkinsonism
- Multiple system atrophy

- Multiple system atrophy
- Vascular parkinsonism
- Corticobasal degeneration

- Vascular parkinsonism

Neuroimaging may show suggestive changes

FIGURE 7.2 — Essential Tremor

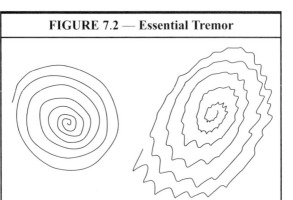

Shown here are Archimedes spirals, drawn from inside outward with at least five turns, produced by a healthy control subject *(left)* and a patient with essential tremor *(right)*.

Bain PG. *Assessing Tremor Severity.* London, UK: Smith-Gordon and Company Limited; 1993.

such as drug-induced parkinsonism and vascular parkinsonism, can be categorized as secondary parkinsonian disorders. However, recent research supports the emerging classification of neurodegenerative disorders according to their underlying pathogenic mechanisms (**Table 7.6**)[7] (see Chapter 6, *Pathogenesis*). **Table 7.7** displays clinical features that differentiate PD from the most common atypical parkinsonism disorders.[7]

- **Progressive Supranuclear Palsy**
  Progressive supranuclear palsy (PSP), one the tauopathies, is characterized by contracted facial muscles, square-wave jerks, dystonic postures of the neck and shoulders, and a tendency to topple when walking. The diagnosis of PSP can be established in most cases by patients' inability to produce vertical saccades; paralysis of first downward, and then later, upward gaze; and eventually, paralysis of lateral gaze with

TABLE 7.4 — Comparison of Parkinson's Disease and Essential Tremor

	Parkinson's Disease	Essential Tremor
Characteristics		
Family history	Usually negative	Positive in 50%
Alcohol	± Effect	Marked tremor reduction
Medical attention sought	Early in course	Often late in course
Age at onset	Mid-adulthood	Childhood, adulthood, or elderly
Tremor type	Resting	Postural, kinetic
Body part affected	Hands, legs	Hands, head, voice
Disease course	Progressive	Slowly progressive; static for long periods
Bradykinesia, rigidity, postural instability	May be present	Never present
Treatment		
Levodopa	Effective	No effect
Propranolol	May decrease tremor	Effective
Primidone	No effect	Effective

7

TABLE 7.5 — Characterization of Parkinsonism	
Clinical Diagnosis	**N (%)**
Parkinson's disease	5,410 (71.5)
PSP	381 (5.0)
MSA	349 (4.6)
Vascular	265 (3.5)
Drug-induced	227 (4.4)
CBD	143 (3.0)
Hemiparkinsonism-hemiatrophy	81 (1.0)
Gait disorders	187 (2.4)
Other	521 (6.9)

Abbreviations: CBD, corticobasal degeneration; MSA, multiple system atrophy; N, number [of subjects]; PSP, progressive supranuclear palsy.

Based on analysis of a combined database of all new patients evaluated in the Movement Disorders Clinic at Baylor College of Medicine, Houston (n = 4,334) and Columbia-Presbyterian Medical Center, New York (n = 3,230).

Adapted from: Jankovic J, et al. *Arch Neurol.* 2000;57:369-372.

retention of reflex eye movements. Some of the differentiating characteristics of PSP are shown in **Table 7.7**. One pathologically based series found gait instability, paucity of tremor, and poor levodopa response to be features that best differentiate PSP from PD.[8]

PSP is one of the neurofibrillary tangle (NFT) diseases, which also includes Alzheimer's disease (AD) and corticobasal degeneration (see below).[9] The cortical NFTs of PSP appear to be antigenically identical to those of AD, most notably with regard to the presence of abnormally phosphorylated tau protein.[9] Staining with anti-tau antibody greatly aids in their identification. Staining for ubiquitin, a peptide involved in proteolysis and occurring in the NFTs of AD

TABLE 7.6 — Emerging Classification of Neurodegenerative Disorders According to Pathogenic Mechanisms

Classification	Examples
Ubiquitin-proteasome disorders	Parkinson's disease
Synucleinopathies	Parkinson's disease; multiple system atrophy; dementia with Lewy bodies
Tauopathies	Progressive supranuclear palsy; corticobasal degeneration; frontotemporal dementia
Polyglutamine expansion diseases	Huntington's disease; spinocerebellar atrophies
Prion diseases	Jakob-Creutzfeld disease

Adapted from: Jankovic J. In: 14th Annual Course. A Comprehensive Review of Movement Disorders for the Clinical Practitioner. Vol 1. Aspen, Colo; July 30-August 2, 2004:679-799.

7

TABLE 7.7 — Parkinsonism Plus Syndromes: Differential Diagnosis

	PD	PSP	MSA	CBD	DLB
Bradykinesia	+	+	+	+	±
Rigidity	+	+	+	+	+
Gait disturbance	+	+	+	+	+
Tremor	+	–	–	±	–
Ataxia	–	–	±	–	–
Dysautonomia	±	±	+	–	±
Dementia	±	+	–	±	+
Dysarthria/dysphagia	±	+	+	+	±
Dystonia	±	±	–	+	–
Eyelid apraxia	–	+	±	±	–
Limb apraxia	–	–	–	+	±
Motor neuron disease	–	–	±	–	–

Myoclonus	±	−	±	+	±
Neuropathy	−	−	±	−	−
Oculomotor deficit	−	+	±	+	±
Sleep impairment	±	±	±	−	±
Asymmetric findings	+	−	−	+	−
Levodopa response	+	±	±	−	−
Levodopa dyskinesia	+	−	−	−	−
Family history	±	−	−	−	−
Putaminal T–2 hypointensity	−	±	+	−	−
Lewy bodies	+	−	±	±	+

Abbreviations: CBD, corticobasal degeneration; DLB, dementia with Lewy bodies; MSA, multiple system atrophy; PD, Parkinson's disease; PSP, progressive supranuclear palsy.

Adapted from: Jankovic J. In: *14th Annual Course. A Comprehensive Review of Movement Disorders for the Clinical Practitioner.* Vol 1. Aspen, Colo; July 30-August 2, 2004:679–799.

and Lewy bodies in PD, is weak or variable in the NFTs of PSP.[9]

Postmortem examinations have disclosed bilateral loss of neurons and gliosis in the periaqueductal gray matter, the superior colliculus, subthalamic nucleus, red nucleus, globus pallidus, dentate nucleus, pretectal and vestibular nuclei, and to some extent, the oculomotor nucleus. The NFTs are globose (round) or flame-shaped and are composed of filaments.

■ Multiple System Atrophy

Multisystem atrophy (MSA), one of the synucleinopathies, is a sporadic, adult-onset, degenerative disorder characterized pathologically by oligodendroglial cytoplasmic inclusions that are positive for stains of α-synuclein.

This disease has been called striatonigral degeneration (when parkinsonism predominates), Shy-Drager syndrome (when autonomic features predominate), and olivopontocerebellar atrophy (when cerebellar features predominate).[10] We now refer to all of these as MSA, since they have all been found to have these characteristic inclusions.[10]

MSA typically presents in patients who are in their 50s. Ninety percent of patients develop parkinsonism; 50% develop cerebellar features. In men, impotence is the earliest feature of autonomic disturbance. Falls are not as common in the first year of this disease as with PSP (the toppling disease). Other features that suggest this diagnosis include urinary incontinence, cold, dusky hands, inspiratory stridor, myoclonic jerks of the fingers, and the "wheelchair-sign" (ie, permanent use of wheelchair is not common in typical PD). The prognosis is poor, with death occurring on the average 9.5 years from presentation. Magnetic resonance imaging (MRI) abnormalities have been described and positron emission tomography (PET) may be helpful but sometimes cannot distinguish from other forms of parkinsonism. Cardiac abnormalities can be detected by radionucleotide uptake techniques. Also an anal or urethral sphincter electromyograph (EMG) is diagnostic for denervation. These reflect the loss of neurons in Onuf's nucleus.[11]

■ Corticobasal Degeneration

Corticobasal degeneration (CBD) is a tauopathy with striking clinical features, including:

- Marked asymmetry
- Focal rigidity and dystonia with contractures
- Apraxia
- Coarse rest and action tremor
- Cortical myoclonus
- Cortical sensory deficit
- Parkinsonism.

Other features include the "alien limb" phenomenon, a gait disorder, and cognitive involvement. Although sometimes it is difficult to distinguish from PSP, the eye movements are relatively spared. The asymmetry should make one suspicious of this devastating disorder. There is no response at all to levodopa. The diagnosis can be strengthened with glucose PET, which demonstrates the asymmetry. However, the confirmation is at autopsy.

The neuropathology is quite characteristic and includes neuronal degeneration of the cortex as well as basal ganglia. The achromatic inclusions can be seen in the neurons and glia of the cortex and other regions. These are tau-positive with a fine filamentous feature. The neurons in which the inclusions reside are ballooned. Also seen are neuronal loss, astrocytosis, and basophilic inclusions (corticobasal inclusions). The pathological features of this disorder greatly overlap with PSP and Pick's disease. Of great significance is a recent report indicating that PSP and CBD share a common tau haplotype, further blurring the distinctions between these two entities.[12]

■ Dementia With Lewy Bodies

Dementia with Lewy Bodies (DLB), considered by some as a variant of Alzheimer's disease (AD) or an overlap between AD and PD, is now well-recognized as an important clinical entity.[7]

Lewy bodies — eosinophilic inclusion bodies found within the cytoplasm of neurons in the cerebral cortex and limbic system — are composed of proteins derived from neurofilaments as well as α-synuclein and ubiquitin.[13] They are found in a number of disorders, including AD, PD, and certain parkinsonian disorders that present with parkinsonism and dementia. In AD, minor extrapyramidal findings usually are overshadowed by progressive cognitive dysfunction, usually allowing clinical differentiation from PD. DLB accounts for 15% to 20% of cases of dementia and may present with prominent parkinsonism.[14,15]

In many patients with DLB, cognitive changes precede parkinsonism, and unlike AD, cognitive deficits alternate with near-normal performance.[13-15] Thus, fluctuation is an important diagnostic indicator.[13,16] Other common features that distinguish DLB from PD include visual hallucinations and postural hypotension that precede exposure to dopaminergic medications.

A number of pathologic features distinguish DLB from other parkinsonian disorders. In DLB, Lewy bodies are found throughout paralimbic and neocortical structures. In addition, there is a distinctive pattern of ubiquitin and α-synuclein immunoreactive degeneration in keeping with this disease's status as a synucleinopathy.

Consensus guidelines for the clinical diagnosis of DLB have been developed and are[14,15]:
- Progressive cognitive decline that interferes with normal function, attention deficits, im-

paired frontal-cortical skills, and visuospatial ability may be especially prominent.

- The presence of one additional feature is required for a diagnosis of "possible," or two additional features for "probable," DLB. Such features include fluctuating cognition, recurrent visual hallucinations, and parkinsonism.
- Features supporting the diagnosis are repeated falls, syncope, transient loss of consciousness, systematized delusions, and hallucinations.
- Unusual findings include clinical or neuroimaging evidence of stroke or a coexisting disorder that may cause the symptoms.

7

Although these clinical criteria for the diagnosis of DLB are specific, their sensitivity is low.[13] Underdiagnosis (usually misdiagnosis as AD) remains common. Current research is focused on ways to enhance detection of DLB.

Management of DLB can be challenging.[3,13,16] Cholinesterase inhibitors may reduce neuropsychiatric features, such as delusions, apathy, agitation, and hallucinations. Levodopa/carbidopa combinations may be used for treatment of parkinsonism. Neuroleptics should be used with caution in patients with DLB since severe extrapyramidal reactions to many antipsychotic medications are a feature of DLB. If behavioral problems persist, low-dose treatment with certain atypical agents, such as quetiapine, may be effective and tolerated. [17,18]

It is important to note that the US FDA has issued a public health advisory regarding the use of atypical neuroleptics for treatment of behaviorally disorders in elderly patients with dementia. Clinical studies of these drugs in this population have shown a higher mortality rate associated with the use of atypical neuroleptics as compared with patients receiving placebo.

■ Vascular Parkinsonism (VP)

Vascular causes account for 3% to 6% of cases of parkinsonism.[19] VP is a heterogeneous disorder that can mimic idiopathic PD, but likely is a disorder separate from PD associated with vascular disease.[20,21] The gait is wide based, which differs from the narrow-based gait seen in PD. Patients with this form of parkinsonism are more likely to present with gait difficulty than tremor, and more likely to have abrupt onset of symptoms, a history of falls, dementia, corticospinal findings, incontinence, or emotional instability.[21,22] In addition, evidence of neurovascular disease is common, and vascular risk factors may be identified more commonly in patients with suspected VP than those with PD.[23] A recent study suggests that the presence of normal olfactory function may be helpful in distinguishing VP from PD.[24]

Usually there is a stepwise worsening, with poor response to levodopa, and the disease is quite symmetrical. Commonly noted lesions on brain imaging in VP are lacunae, white matter changes consistent with Binswanger's pathology and, rarely, territorial infarcts.[21] Since coincidental vascular lesions are common in idiopathic PD, the mere presence of these lesions on brain imaging is not diagnostic of VP. Hurtig has outlined a set of criteria for this disorder, including a stepwise evolution, the presence of vascular risk factors, and imaging studies with at least two infarcts in the basal ganglia.[25]

■ Postencephalitic Parkinsonism

Exposure to an infectious agent, such as the one (or more) responsible for the 1917-1928 pandemic of encephalitis lethargica, was once thought to be a primary cause of PD.[7] About 40% of the affected individuals died during the acute illness, and parkinsonism developed in 50% of the survivors within 5 years and 80% within 10 years. However, since no definite instance of encephalitis lethargica has been recorded since 1930, it is safe to say that postencephalitic parkinsonism has disappeared. Rarely, a Parkinson-like syndrome has been described associated with other forms of encephalitis, particularly that due to Japanese B virus.

■ **Normal-Pressure Hydrocephalus**

Normal-pressure hydrocephalus (NPH) can create a Parkinson-like condition, with gait and postural instability and, at times, bradykinesia. The gait and parkinsonian features associated with NPH include short steps, wide base, stiff legs, start hesitation, and freezing.[7] In addition, NPH patients may exhibit cognitive decline and urinary incontinence and may later develop PD. Shunting may be considered in selected patients with NPH.[7]

■ **Drug-Induced Parkinsonism**

Many drugs can induce parkinsonism.[26] Although the antipsychotic agents (**Table 7.8**) are well recognized in this regard, various others medications (**Table 7.9**) may also induce parkinsonism.[26]

Drug-induced parkinsonism may be clinically indistinguishable from Parkinson's disease. Akinesia, rigidity, postural abnormalities, and tremor may be present. Bradykinesia is the earliest, most common, and often the only manifestation, accounting for the expressionless face, loss of associated movements, slow initiation of motor activity, and disturbed speech. Rigidity of the extremities, neck, or trunk, usually without a "cogwheel" phenomenon, may occur after the onset of bradykinesia. Although the characteristic parkinsonian "pill-rolling" tremor at rest may be present, postural tremor resembling essential tremor may also be seen.

Drug-induced parkinsonism may be differentiated from PD by certain characteristics (**Table 7.10**).

TABLE 7.8 — Neuroleptics and Related Agents

Trade Name	Generic Name
Phenothiazines	
Compazine	Prochlorperazine
Etrafon, Triavil	Perphenazine and amitriptyline
Levoprome	Methotrimeprazine
Mellaril	Thioridazine
Phenergan	Promethazine
Prolixin	Fluphenazine
Norzine, Torecan	Thiethylperazine
Serentil	Mesoridazine
Sparine	Promazine
Stelazine	Trifluoperazine
Thorazine	Chlorpromazine
Trilafon	Perphenazine
Butyrophenones	
Haldol	Haloperidol
Fentanyl	Droperidol
Thioxanthenes	
Navane	Thiothixene
Taractan	Chlorprothixene
Benzamide	
Reglan	Metoclopramide
Dihydroindolone	
Moban	Molindone
Dibenzoxazepine	
Loxitane	Loxapine
Dibenzodiazepine	
Clozaril	Clozapine
Seroquel	Quetiapine
Benzisoxazole	
Risperdal	Risperidone
Thienobenzodiazepine	
Zyprexa	Olanzapine
Seroquel	Quetiapine

Continued

Others	
Abilify	Aripiprazole
Geodon	Ziprasodone
Zofran	Ondansetron

Adapted from: Watts RL, Koller WC, eds. *Movement Disorders: Neurologic Principles and Practice*. 2nd ed. New York, NY: The McGraw-Hill Companies; 2004:395.

TABLE 7.9 — Miscellaneous Drugs Associated With Parkinsonism

- Reserpine
- Tetrabenazine
- α-Methyldopa
- Calcium-channel blockers:
  - Cinnarizine
  - Flunarizine
- Amiodarone
- Bethanechol
- Pyridostigmine
- Lithium
- Diazepam
- Selective serotonin reuptake inhibitors:
  - Fluoxetine
  - Paroxetine
  - Sertraline
- Phenelzine
- Procaine
- Meperidine
- Amphotericin B
- Cephaloridine
- 5-Fluorouracil
- Doxorubicin hydrochloride
- "Ecstasy"

Adapted from: Watts RL, Koller WC, eds. *Movement Disorders: Neurologic Principles and Practice*. 2nd ed. New York, NY: The McGraw-Hill Companies; 2004:399.

Although a number of approaches to preclinical detection of PD have been investigated, a practical, inexpensive, sensitive, specific screening test has yet to be made available. Furthermore, in the absence of a disease-specific biologic marker, a definitive diagnosis of PD can be made only at autopsy. (Two separate pathological studies concluded that only 76% of clinically diagnosed Parkinson's patients actually met the pathologic criteria; 24% had other causes of parkinsonism.[27])

Neuroimaging techniques have evolved considerably over just the past few decades. It is now technically possible to perform functional imaging of the dopaminergic system to identify abnormalities early in PD, to assess neuronal degeneration, and potentially to monitor progression and as well the effect of treatment.[28-31]

The four main approaches to functional imaging are: magnetic resonance imaging (MRI); positron emission tomography (PET); single photon emission tomography (SPECT); and magnetic resonance spectroscopy (MRS).

■ Magnetic Resonance Imaging (MRI)

MRI is most useful in assessing structural changes in the dopaminergic system, particularly the substantia nigra.[32,33] Several studies have found MRI useful in differentiating between PD and atypical parkinsonian syndromes.[33-36] MRI also can detect activation-induced changes in oxygenation of venous blood draining from specific brain regions when subjects perform tasks (the BOLD technique).[30] Although MRI remains an important research tool, its use in clinical practice is limited.

■ Positron Emission Tomography (PET)

PET imaging provides the means to study neurochemical, hemodynamic, or metabolic processes that

TABLE 7.10 — Clinical Features That May Distinguish Drug-Induced Parkinsonism From Idiopathic Parkinson's Disease		
	Drug-Induced Parkinsonism	Idiopathic Parkinson's Disease
Symptom onset	Bilateral and symmetric	Unilateral or asymmetrical
Course	Acute or subacute	Insidious, chronic
Tremor type	Bilateral or symmetric postur or rest tremor	Unilateral or symmetric rest tremor
Anticholinergic drug response	May be pronounced	Usually mild to moderate
Withdrawal of offending drug	Remittance typically within weeks to months	Symptoms and signs slowly progress

Adapted from: Watts RL, Koller WC, eds. *Movement Disorders: Neurologic Principles and Practice.* 2nd ed. New York, NY: The McGraw-Hill Companies; 2004:396.

underlie PD and other movement disorders.[28-31] PET imaging has contributed significantly to insights into the nigrostriatal dopamine system and its role in the pathophysiology of PD. Clinically, fluorodopa/PET has provided a way to assess the integrity of the striatal dopaminergic terminals. Characteristic reduction of fluorodopa uptake, particularly in the putamen, can be demonstrated in virtually all patients with PD, even in the early stages. Impairment of uptake in an asymptomatic, clinically normal member of a kindred in which five of 10 adult siblings developed apparent PD suggested a subclinical defect in the presynaptic nigrostriatal system.[37]

At onset of symptoms, PD patients have shown a 30% loss of putamen [^{18}F] dopa uptake. Unfortunately, [^{18}F] dopa PET does not differentiate between PD and atypical parkinsonisms. However, ^{18}F-fluorodeoxyglucose (FDG) and PET show consistent reduced resting levels of striatal glucose metabolism in atypical parkinsonism. This contrasts with PD in which this is normal or elevated. In a recent study of parkinsonism associated with the α-synuclein gene, PET findings were identical to those of idiopathic PD.[38]

[^{18}F] dopa PET provides a means of objectively monitoring progression of disease, as well as an objective demonstration of function of fetal mesencephalic tissue implants.

■ **Single Photon Emission Computed Tomography**
Ligands have now become available for imaging the presynaptic and postsynaptic system by single photon emission computed tomography (SPECT), which could potentially contribute to the differential diagnosis between parkinson-plus syndromes and PD.[39] Striatal binding to the presynaptic dopamine transporter of the cocaine derivative [^{123}I] β-CIT, also known as DOPASCAN, was significantly diminished contralateral to both the clinically affected and unaffected side

in hemiparkinsonian patients.[40] Binding was also significantly decreased in comparison to age-expected values ranging from 36% in Hoehn and Yahr stage I to 71% in stage V.

In a recent study, Jennings and associates performed [^{123}I] β-CIT uptake studies in 35 patients referred by community neurologists with a diagnosis of suspected PD.[41] They found that SPECT imaging at referral appeared to be a useful tool of identify patients were thought to have PD but who, after 6 months' follow up, do not have PD. It is now possible to visualize and quantify the degeneration of striatal neurons in parkinsonism, but it is not always possible to distinguish between them.[42]

Thus imaging of presynaptic dopamine transporters using this or other new ligands may prove to be useful in early detection of individuals at risk. In fact, SPECT's potential as a screening method for early or even presymptomatic PD seems to have become a practical reality.[39,41] The technique's potential as an objective method of monitoring the efficacy of new pharmacologic therapies is currently being studied.

The promise of this approach is enhanced by the relative simplicity, availability, and lower cost of SPECT compared with the other neuroimaging techniques.

■ Magnetic Resonance Spectroscopy (MRS)

MRS provides a noninvasive, *in vivo* insight into brain metabolism by quantifying concentrations of basal ganglia and cerebral cortex metabolites such as N-acetylaspartate (NAA), choline (Cho), and creatine (Cr). Although several small studies found that MRS may be useful in differentiating parkinsonian syndromes, the results were not consistent.[43-45] While MRS is a valuable research tool, its clinical utility is limited due to its lower sensitivity and special resolution as compared with radionuclide PET and SPECT imaging.[30]

■ **Other Emerging Techniques**

Transcranial ultrasound has been suggested as a novel and convenient imaging technique potentially useful in differentiating idiopathic PD from atypical parkinsonian syndromes. A recent study in 102 patients with PD, 34 patients with MSA, and 21 patients with PSP, found that increased echogenicity of the substantia nigra was predictive of PD, whereas a low echogenic substantia nigra, combined with a hyperechogenic lentiform nucleus, strongly suggested an atypical parkinsonian syndrome.[46]

Clinical evaluation of patients with a disease such as PD, with its multiple signs and symptoms that differ in presence and intensity among patients, is a complex, often difficult endeavor. Evaluation can be quantitative, with measurements in objective physical units, or qualitative, using subjective scales to assess symptoms and signs and/or functional disability. Quantitative testing, with its often time-consuming methods and expensive or sophisticated equipment, is not generally used to assess and follow patients with PD. Nor is it useful in the evaluation of the large number of patients involved in clinical trials.

Qualitative testing, on the other hand, is relatively rapid and simple and is generally used by neurologists in the staging, evaluation, and following of Parkinson patients. A number of rating scales, with a somewhat standardized core of assessment and a four-point scoring system, have been designed. One of the most widely used, the Unified Parkinson's Disease Rating Scale (UPDRS), assesses 42 items, scored from 0 to 4, to establish individual patients' mental status, activities of daily living, motor function, and complications of therapy (**Table 7.11**). The UPDRS is often accompanied by a Step-Second Test (**Table 7.12**) and the Schwab and England Activities of Daily Living Scale (**Table 7.13**).

REFERENCES

1. Paulson HL, Stern MB. Clinical manifestations of Parkinson's disease. In: Watts RL, Koller WC, eds. *Movement Disorders: Neuroloogic Principles and Practice.* 2nd ed. New York, NY: The McGraw-Hill Companies; 2004:233-245.

2. Gelb DJ, Oliver E, Gilman S. Diagnostic criteria for Parkinson's disease. *Arch Neurol.* 1999;56:33-39.

3. Christine CW, Aminoff MJ. Clinical differentiation of parkinsonian syndromes: prognostic and therapeutic relevance. *Am J Med.* 2004;117:412-419.

4. Louis ED. Essential tremor. *Lancet Neurol.* 2005;4:100-110.

5. Sullivan KL, Hauser RA, Zesiewicz TA. Essential tremor. Epidemiology, diagnosis, and treatment. *Neurologist.* 2004;10:250-258.

6. Jankovic J, Rajput AH, McDermott MP, Perl DP. The evolution of diagnosis in early Parkinson disease. Parkinson Study group. *Arch Neurol.* 2000;57:369-372.

7. Jankovic J. Parkinsonism plus syndromes and secondary parkinsonian disorders. In: 14th Annual Course. A Comprehensive Review of Movement Disorders for the Clinical Practitioner. Vol 1. Aspen, Colo; July 30-August 2, 2004:679-799.

8. Litvan I, Campbell G, Mangone CA, et al. Which clinical features differentiate progressive supranuclear palsy (Steele-Richardson-Olszewski syndrome) from related disorders? A clinicopathological study. *Brain.* 1997;120:65-74.

9. Golbe LI. Progressive supranuclear palsy (Richardson's disease). In: Watts RL, Koller WC, eds. *Movement Disorders: Neurologic Principles and Practice.* 2nd ed. New York, NY: The McGraw-Hill Companies; 2004:339-358.

10. Shulman LM, Minagar A, Weiner WJ. Multiple-system atrophy. In: Watts RL, Koller WC, eds. *Movement Disorders: Neurologic Principles and Practice.* 2nd ed. New York, NY: The McGraw-Hill Companies; 2004:359-369.

7

TABLE 7.11 — Unified Parkinson's Disease Rating Scale (UPDRS)

Mentation, Behavior and Mood

Intellectual Impairment

0= None.

1= Mild. Consistent forgetfulness with partial recollection of events and no other difficulties.

2= Moderate memory loss, with disorientation and moderate difficulty handling complex problems. Mild but definite impairment of function at home with need of occasional prompting.

3= Severe memory loss with disorientation for time and often for place. Severe impairment in handling problems.

4= Severe memory loss with orientation preserved to person only. Unable to make judgments or solve problems. Requires much help with personal care. Cannot be left alone at all.

Thought Disorder (Due to dementia or drug intoxication)

0= None.

1= Vivid dreaming.

2= "Benign" hallucinations with insight retained.

3= Occasional to frequent hallucinations or delusions; without insight; could interfere with daily activities.

4= Persistent hallucinations, delusions, or florid psychosis. Not able to care for self.

Depression

0= Not present.

1= Periods of sadness or guilt greater than normal, never sustained for days or weeks.

2= Sustained depression (1 week or more).

3= Sustained depression with vegetative symptoms (insomnia, anorexia, weight loss, loss of interest).

4= Sustained depression with vegetative symptoms and suicidal thoughts or intent.

Motivation/Initiative

0= Normal.

1= Less assertive than usual, more passive.

2= Loss of initiative or disinterest in elective (nonroutine) activities.

3= Loss of initiative or disinterest in day-to-day (routine) activities.

4= Withdrawn, complete loss of motivation.

Continued

Activities of Daily Living
(Determine for "On"/"Off")

Speech
0= Normal.
1= Mildly affected; no difficulty being understood.
2= Moderately affected; sometimes asked to repeat statements.
3= Severely affected; frequently asked to repeat statements.
4= Unintelligible most of the time.

Salivation
0= Normal.
1= Slight but definite excess of saliva in mouth; may experience nighttime drooling.
2= Moderately excessive saliva; may experience minimal drooling.
3= Marked excess of saliva with some drooling.
4= Marked drooling, constantly requires tissue or handkerchief.

Swallowing
0= Normal.
1= Rare choking.
2= Occasional choking.
3= Requires soft food.
4= Requires nasogastric tube or gastrotomy feeding.

Handwriting
0= Normal.
1= Slightly slow or small.
2= Moderately slow or small; all words are legible.
3= Severely affected; not all words are legible.
4= The majority of words are not legible.

Cutting Food and Handling Utensils
0= Normal.
1= Somewhat slow and clumsy, but no help needed.
2= Can cut most foods, although clumsy and slow; some help needed.
3= Food must be cut by someone, but can still feed self slowly.
4= Needs to be fed.

Dressing
0= Normal.
1= Somewhat slow, but no help needed.
2= Occasional assistance with buttoning, getting arms into sleeves.
3= Considerable help required, but can do some things alone.
4= Helpless.

Continued

Hygiene
0= Normal.
1= Somewhat slow, but no help needed.
2= Needs help to shower or bathe; very slow in hygienic care.
3= Requires assistance for washing, brushing teeth, combing hair, using the toilet.
4= Helpless (Foley catheter or other mechanical aids needed).

Turning in Bed and Adjusting Bed Clothes
0= Normal.
1= Somewhat slow and clumsy, but no help needed.
2= Can turn alone or adjust sheets, but with great difficulty.
3= Can initiate movement, but not turn or adjust sheets alone.
4= Helpless.

Falling (Unrelated to Freezing)
0= None.
1= Rare falling.
2= Occasionally falls, less than once per day.
3= Falls an average of once daily.
4= Falls more than once daily.

Freezing When Walking
0= None.
1= Rare freezing when walking; may have start-hesitation.
2= Occasional freezing when walking.
3= Frequent freezing; occasionally falls due to freezing.
4= Frequent falls due to freezing.

Walking
0= Normal.
1= Mild difficulty; may not swing arms or may tend to drag leg.
2= Moderate difficulty, but requires little or no assistance.
3= Cannot walk at all, even with assistance.

Tremor
0= Absent.
1= Slight and infrequently present.
2= Moderate; bothersome to patient.
3= Severe; interferes with many activities.
4= Marked; interferes with most activities.

Sensory Complaints Related to Parkinsonism
0= None.
1= Occasionally has numbness, tingling, or mild aching.
2= Frequently has numbness, tingling, or aching; not distressing.
3= Frequent painful sensations.
4= Excruciating pain.

Continued

Motor Examination
(Determine for "On"/"Off")

Speech

0= Normal.
1= Slight loss of expression, diction and/or volume.
2= Monotone, slurred but understandable; moderately impaired.
3= Marked impairment, difficult to understand.
4= Unintelligible.

Facial Expression

0= Normal.
1= Slight hypomimia, could be normal "poker face."
2= Slight but definitely abnormal diminution of facial expression.
3= Moderate hypomimia; lips parted some of the time.
4= Masked or fixed facies with severe or complete loss of facial expression; lips parted $1/4$ inch or more.

Tremor at Rest

0= Absent.
1= Slight and infrequently present.
2= Mild in amplitude and persistent; or, moderate in amplitude but only intermittently present.
3= Moderate in amplitude and present most of the time.
4= Marked in amplitude and present most of the time.

Action or Postural Tremor of Hands

0= Absent.
1= Slight; present with action.
2= Moderate in amplitude; present with action.
3= Moderate in amplitude with posture holding as well as action.
4= Marked in amplitude; interferes with feeding.

Rigidity (Judged on passive movement of major joints with patient relaxed in sitting position. Cogwheeling to be ignored.)

0= Absent.
1= Slight or detectable only when activated by mirror or other movements.
2= Mild to moderate.
3= Marked, but full range of motion easily achieved.
4= Severe, range of motion achieved with difficulty.

Continued

Finger Taps (Patient taps thumb with index finger in rapid succession with widest amplitude possible, each hand separately.)

0= Normal ($\geq 15/5$ seconds).

1= Mild slowing and/or reduction in amplitude (11-14/5 seconds).

2= Moderately impaired. Definite and early fatiguing. May have occasional arrests in movement (7-10/5 seconds).

3= Severely impaired. Frequent hesitation in initiating movements or arrests in ongoing movement (3-6/5 seconds).

4= Can barely perform the task (0-2/5 seconds).

Hand Movements (Patient opens and closes hands in rapid succession with widest amplitude possible, each hand separately.)

0= Normal.

1= Mild slowing and/or reduction in amplitude.

2= Moderately impaired. Definite and early fatiguing. May have occasional arrests in movement.

3= Severely impaired. Frequent hesitation in initiating movements or arrests in ongoing movement.

4= Can barely perform the task.

Rapid Alternating Movements of Hands (Pronation-supination movements of hands, vertically or horizontally, with as large an amplitude as possible, both hands simultaneously.)

0= Normal.

1= Mild slowing and/or reduction in amplitude.

2= Moderately impaired. Definite and early fatiguing. May have occasional arrests in movement.

3= Severely impaired. Frequent hesitation in initiating movements or arrests in ongoing movement.

4= Can barely perform the task.

Leg Agility (With knee bent, patient taps heel on ground in rapid succession, picking up entire leg. Amplitude should be about 3 inches.)

0= Normal.

1= Mild slowing and/or reduction in amplitude.

2= Moderately impaired. Definite and early fatiguing. May have occasional arrests in movement.

3= Severely impaired. Frequent hesitation in initiating movements or arrests in ongoing movement.

4= Can barely perform the task.

Continued

Rising From Chair (Patient attempts to arise from a straight-back wood or metal chair, with arms folded across chest.)
0= Normal.
1= Slow; or may need more than one attempt.
2= Pushes self up from arms of seat.
3= Tends to fall back and may have to try more than 1 time, but can get up without help.
4= Unable to rise without help.

Posture
0= Normal erect.
1= Not quite erect, slightly stooped posture; could be normal for older person.
2= Moderately stooped posture, definitely abnormal; can be slightly leaning to one side.
3= Severely stooped posture with kyphosis; can be moderately leaning to one side.
4= Marked flexion with extreme abnormality of posture.

Gait
0= Normal.
1= Walks slowly, may shuffle with short steps, but no festination or propulsion.
2= Walks with difficulty, but requires little or no assistance; may have some festination, short steps, or propulsion.
3= Severe disturbance of gait, requiring assistance.
4= Cannot walk at all, even with assistance.

Postural Stability (Response to sudden posterior displacement produced by pull on shoulders while patient is erect, with eyes open and feet slightly apart. Patient is prepared.)
0= Normal.
1= Retropulsion, but recovers unaided.
2= Absence of postural response; would fall if not caught by examiner.
3= Very unstable, tends to lose balance spontaneously.
4= Unable to stand without assistance.

Body Bradykinesia and Hypokinesia (Combining slowness, hesitancy, decreased arm swing, small amplitude, and poverty of movement in general.)
0= None.
1= Minimal slowness, giving movement a deliberate character; could be normal for some persons. Possibly reduced amplitude.
2= Mild degree of slowness and poverty of movement that is definitely abnormal. Alternatively, some reduced amplitude.
3= Moderate slowness, poverty or small amplitude of movement.
4= Marked slowness, poverty or small amplitude of movement.

Complications of Therapy
(Within the past week)

Dyskinesias
Duration: *What proportion of the walking day are dyskinesias present?* (Historical information)
0= None.
1= 1% to 25% of day.
2= 26% to 50% of day.
3= 51% to 75% of day.
4= 76% to 100% of day.

Disability: *How disabling are the dyskinesias?* (Historical information; may be modified by office examination)
0= Not disabling.
1= Mildly disabling.
2= Moderately disabling.
3= Severely disabling.
4= Completely disabled.

Painful Dyskinesias: *How painful are the dyskinesias?*
0= No painful dyskinesias.
1= Slight.
2= Moderate.
3= Severe.
4= Marked.

Presence of Early Morning Dystonia (Historical information)
0= No
1= Yes

Clinical Fluctuations
Are any "off" periods predictable as to timing after a dose of medication?
0= No
1= Yes

Are any "off" periods unpredictable as to timing after a dose of medication?
0= No
1= Yes

Do any of the "off" periods come on suddenly (eg, over a few seconds)?
0= No
1= Yes

Continued

What proportion of the walking day is the patient "off" on average?
 0= None.
 1= 1% to 25% of day.
 2= 26% to 50% of day.
 3= 51% to 75% of day.
 4= 76% to 100% of day.

Other Complications

Does the patient have anorexia, nausea, or vomiting?
 0= No
 1= Yes

Does the patient have any sleep disturbances (eg, insomnia or hypersomnolence)?
 0= No
 1= Yes

Does the patient have symptomatic orthostasis?
 0= No
 1= Yes

Record the patient's blood pressure, pulse, and weight on the scoring form.

Modified Hoehn and Yahr Staging

Stage 0   = No signs of disease.
Stage 1   = Unilateral disease.
Stage 1.5 = Unilateral plus axial involvement.
Stage 2   = Bilateral disease, without impairment of balance.
Stage 2.5 = Mild bilateral disease, with recovery on pull test.
Stage 3   = Mild to moderate bilateral disease; some postural instability; physically independent.
Stage 4   = Severe disability; still able to talk or stand unassisted.
Stage 5   = Wheelchair bound or bedridden unless aided.

TABLE 7.12 — Step-Second Test

- *Steps Score*: number of steps with right foot per round trip of 15 feet out plus 15 feet back

- *Second Score*: number of seconds per round trip of 15 feet out plus 15 feet back

- *Scoring*:
  0 = Not disabling
  1 = Mildly disabling
  2 = Moderately disabling
  3 = Severely disabling
  4 = Completely disabled

11. Quinn N. Multiple system atrophy—how do you really diagnose it? American Academy of Neurology. 53rd Annual Meeting. Education Program Syllabus. Philadelphia, Pa; May 5-11, 2001:64-75.

12. Houlden H, Baker M, Morris HR, et al. Corticobasal degeneration and progressive supranuclear palsy share a common tau haplotype. *Neurology*. 2001;56:1702-1706.

13. Geldmacher DS. Dementia with Lewy bodies: diagnosis and clinical approach. *Clev Clin J Med.* 2004;71:789-790, 792-794, 797-798.

14. McKeith IG, Galasko D, Kosaka K, et al. Consensus guidelines for the clinical and pathologic diagnosis of dementia with Lewy bodies (DLB): report of the consortium on DLB international workshop. *Neurology.* 1996;47:1113-1124.

15. McKeith IG, Ballard GG, Perry RH, et al. Prospective validation of consensus criteria for the diagnosis of dementia with Lewy bodies. *Neurology*. 2000;54:1050-1058.

16. Frank C. Dementia with Lewy bodies. Review of diagnosis and pharmacologic management. *Can Fam Physician.* 2003; 49:1304-1311.

17. Swanberg MM, Cummings JL. Benefit-risk considerations in the treatment of dementia with Lewy bodies. *Drug Saf.* 2002;25:511-523.

TABLE 7.13 — Schwab and England Activities of Daily Living Scale

100% ...... Completely independent. Able to do all chores without slowness, difficulty, or impairment. Essentially normal. Unaware of any difficulty.

90% ...... Completely independent. Able to do all chores with some degree of slowness, difficulty, and impairment. Might take twice as long. Beginning to be aware of difficulty.

80% ...... Completely independent in most chores. Takes twice as long. Conscious of difficulty and slowness.

70% ...... Not completely independent. More difficulty with some chores than others. Takes 3 to 4 times as long to complete some chores. Must spend a large part of the day with chores.

60% ...... Some dependency. Can do most chores, but exceedingly slowly and with much effort. Makes errors; some chores impossible.

50% ...... More dependent. Help with half the chores, slower, etc. Difficulty with everything.

40% ...... Very dependent. Can assist with all chores, but can do few alone.

30% ...... With effort, now and then does a few chores alone or begins alone. Much help needed.

20% ...... Nothing alone. Can be a slight help with some chores. Severe invalid.

10% ...... Totally dependent, helpless. Complete invalid.

0% ...... Vegetative, functions such as swallowing, bladder, and bowel functions are not functioning. Bedridden.

18. Fernandez HH, Trieschmann ME, Burke MA, Friedman JH. Quetiapine for psychosis in Parkinson's disease vs dementia with Lewy bodies. *J Clin Psychiatry.* 2002;63:513-515.

19. Foltynie T, Barker R, Brayne C. Vascular parkinsonism: a review of the precision and frequency of the diagnosis. *Neuroepidemiology.* 2002;21:1-7.

20. Sibon I, Fenelon G, Quinn NP, Tison F. Vascular parkinsonism. *J Neurol.* 2004;251:513-524.

21. Thanvi B, Lo N, Robinson T. Vascular parkinsonism—an important cause of parkinsonism in older people. *Age Ageing.* 2005;34:114-119.

22. Winikates J, Jankovic J. Clinical correlates of vascular parkinsonism. *Arch Neurol.* 1999;56:98-102.

23. Demirkiran M, Bozdemir H, Sarcia Y. Vascular parkinsonism: a distinct, heterogeneous clinical entity. *Acta Neurol Scand.* 2001;104:63-67.

24. Katzenschlager R, Zijlmans J, Evans A, Watt H, Lees AJ. Olfactory function distinguishes vascular parkinsonism from Parkinson's disease. *J Neurol Neurosurg Psychiatry.* 2004; 75:1749-1752.

25. Hurtig HI. Vascular parkinsonism. In: Stern MB, Koller WC, eds. *Parkinsonian Syndromes.* New York, NY: Marcel Dekker; 1992:81-93.

26. Hubble JP. Drug-induced parkinsonism. In: Watts RL, Koller WC, eds. *Movement Disorders: Neurologic Principles and Practice.* 2nd ed. New York, NY: The McGraw-Hill Companies; 2004:395-402.

27. Hughes AJ, Daniel SE, Kilford L, Lees AJ. Accuracy of clinical diagnosis of idiopathic Parkinson's disease: a clinicopathological study of 100 cases. *J Neurol Neurosurg Psychiatry.* 1992;55:181-184.

28. Bohnen NI, Frey KA. The role of positron emission tomography in movement disorders. *Neuroimaging Clin N Am.* 2003;13:791-803.

29. Antonini A, DeNotaris R. PET and SPECT functional imaging in Parkinson's disease. *Sleep Med.* 2004;5:201-206.

30. Brooks DJ. Neuroimaging of movement disorders. In: Watts RL, Koller WC, eds. *Movement Disorders: Neurologic Principles and Practice.* 2nd ed. New York, NY: The McGraw-Hill Companies; 2004:35-57.

31. Kemp PM. Imaging the dopaminergic system in suspected parkinsonism, drug induced movement disorders, Lewy body dementia. *Nucl Med Commun.* 2005;26:87-96.

32. Hutchinson M, Raff U. Structural changes of the substantia nigra in Parkinson's disease as revealed by MR imaging. *Am J Neuroradiol.* 2000;21:697-701.

33. Schrag JB, Good CD, Miszkiel K,et al. Differentiation of atypical parkinsonian syndromes with routine MRI. *Neurology.* 2000;54:697-702.

34. Schulz JB, Skalej M, Wedekind D, et al. Magnetic resonance imaging-based volumetry differentiates idiopathic Parkinson's syndrome from multiple system atropy and progressive supranuclear palsy. *Ann Neurol.* 1999;45:65-74.

35. Schrag A, Kingsley D, Phatouros C, et al. Clinical usefulness of magnetic resonance imaging in multiple system atrophy. *J Neurol Neurosurg Psychiatry.* 1998;65:65-71.

36. Kraft E, Schwarz J, Trenkwalder C, Vogl T, Pfluger T, Oertel WH. The combination of hypointense and hyperintense signal changes on T_2-weighted magnetic resonance imaging sequences: a specific marker of multiple system atrophy? *Arch Neurol.* 1999;56:225-228.

37. Sawle GV, Wroe SJ, Lees AJ, Brooks DJ, Frackowiak RS. The identification of presymptomatic parkinsonism: clinical and [18F]dopa positron emission tomography studies in an Irish kindred. *Ann Neurol.* 1992;32:609-617.

38. Samii A, Markopoulou K, Wszolek ZK, et al. PET studies of parkinsonism associated with mutation in the alpha-synuclein gene. *Neurology.* 1999;53:2097-2102.

7

39. Tissingh G, Booij J, Winogrodzka A, van Royen EA, Wolters EC. IBZM- and CIT-SPECT of the dopaminergic system in parkinsonism. *J Neural Transm.* 1997;50(suppl):31-37.

40. Asenbaum S, Brucke T, Pirker W, et al. Imaging of dopamine transporters with iodine-123-beta-CIT and SPECT in Parkinson's disease. *J Nucl Med.* 1997;38:1-6.

41. Jennings DL, Seibyl JP, Oakes D, Eberly S, Murphy J, Marek K. (123I) beta-CIT and single-photon emission computed tomography vs clinical evaluation in Parkinson syndrome: unmasking an early diagnosis. *Arch Neurol.* 2004;61:1224-1229.

42. Parkinson Study Group. A multicenter assessment of dopamine transporter imaging with DOPASCAN/SPECT in parkinsonism. *Neurology.* 2000;55:1540-1547.

43. Federico F, Simone IL, Lucivero V, et al. Usefulness of proton magnetic resonance spectroscopy in differentiating parkinsonian syndromes. *Ital J Neurol Sci.* 1999;20:223-229.

44. Clarke CE, Lowry M. Systematic review of proton magnetic resonance spectroscopy on the striatum in parkinsonian syndromes. *Eur J Neurol.* 2001;8:573-577.

45. Firbank MJ, Harrison RM, O'Brien JT. A comprehensive review of proton magnetic resonance spectroscopy studies in dementia and Parkinson's disease. *Dement Geriatr Cogn Disord.* 2002;14:64-76.

46. Behnke S, Berg D, Naumann M, Becker G. Differentiation of Parkinson's disease and atypical parkinsonian syndromes by transcranial ultrasound. *J Neurol Neurosurg Psychiatry.* 2005;76:423-425.

8 Treatment

The pharmacologic/surgical treatment of Parkinson's disease (PD) can be divided into three major conceptual categories:

- Symptomatic, to improve signs and symptoms of the disease
- Neuroprotective, to interfere with the pathophysiologic mechanisms of the disease
- Restorative, to provide new neurons or to stimulate growth and function of remaining cells (see Chapter 11, *Surgery*).

Although the goal of therapy is to reverse the functional disability, abolition of all symptoms and signs is not currently possible even with high doses of current medications. Therefore, the long-term goal in treating PD is to keep the patient functioning independently for as long as possible.[1] Furthermore, treatment must be highly individualized (a retired patient may require less control than one who is still working, for example), and the patient, as well as the physician, plays a major role in therapeutic decisions.

The treatment of PD with levodopa has been called one of the success stories of modern medicine.[2] The precursor of dopamine in the catecholamine synthetic chain, it can be taken orally because it crosses the blood-brain barrier, whereas dopamine does not.[3] When first introduced in the 1960s, the new drug's dramatic results in even severely affected Parkinson patients raised the hope that all neurodegenerative diseases might be treated with replacement of depleted transmitters. But complications of chronic therapy soon became apparent, superimposing upon the disease-related problems an additional burden of motor fluctuations (the "on-off" reaction), dyskinesias, and visual hallucinations.

Although levodopa has remained the most effective drug available for the relief of symptoms in PD, six additional and distinctly different pharmacologic advances during the last 3 decades have significantly augmented the antiparkinson armamentarium:

- Carbidopa, an inhibitor of dopa decarboxylase, which, combined with levodopa, reduces peripheral decarboxylation of levodopa to dopamine
- Controlled release carbidopa/levodopa to prolong levodopa's 90-minute half-life
- Dopamine agonists, sometimes used as pharmacologically active substitutes for carbidopa/levodopa in early disease and to provide supplementation in later stages
- Inhibitors of catechol-O-methyltransferase (COMT) to increase the amount of levodopa crossing the blood-brain barrier
- Monoamine oxidase type B (MAO-B) inhibitors to slow dopamine's metabolic breakdown.
- N-methyl-D-aspartate (NMDA) receptor antagonist amantadine to reduce dyskinesia.

The initial decision in the management of PD is whether any pharmacotherapy is needed.[1-3] There is no conclusive evidence that treatment is helpful before symptoms start to affect the patient's life. Eventually PD progresses, however, and symptomatic treatment becomes necessary. The decision is usually made on the basis of how symptoms are affecting individual patients and whether they interfere with a job or with the ability to handle domestic, financial, or social affairs. An algorithm for the progressive treatment of PD is seen in **Figure 8.1**.[4]

FIGURE 8.1 — Options in Managing Parkinson's Disease

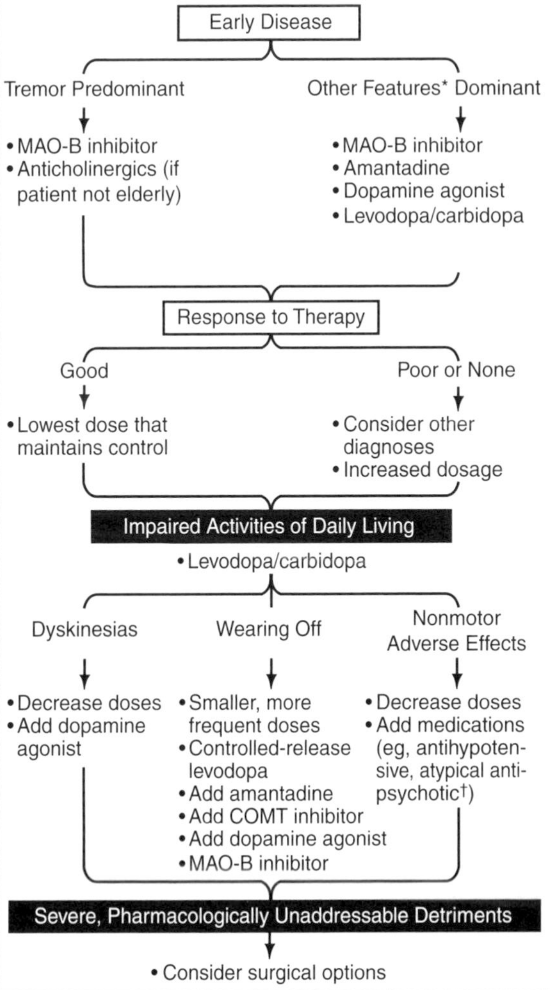

Early Disease

Tremor Predominant
- MAO-B inhibitor
- Anticholinergics (if patient not elderly)

Other Features* Dominant
- MAO-B inhibitor
- Amantadine
- Dopamine agonist
- Levodopa/carbidopa

Response to Therapy

Good
- Lowest dose that maintains control

Poor or None
- Consider other diagnoses
- Increased dosage

Impaired Activities of Daily Living
- Levodopa/carbidopa

Dyskinesias
- Decrease doses
- Add dopamine agonist

Wearing Off
- Smaller, more frequent doses
- Controlled-release levodopa
- Add amantadine
- Add COMT inhibitor
- Add dopamine agonist
- MAO-B inhibitor

Nonmotor Adverse Effects
- Decrease doses
- Add medications (eg, antihypotensive, atypical antipsychotic†)

Severe, Pharmacologically Unaddressable Detriments
- Consider surgical options

Abbreviations: COMT, catechol-*O*-methyltransferase; MAO-B, monoamine oxidase B.

* Rigidity, bradykinesia, akinesia, impaired postural reflexes.
† Quetiapine, clozapine.

Once patient and physician have decided to proceed with treatment, the choice is whether to introduce levodopa or another antiparkinsonian agent. All patients are likely to develop complications associated with long-term use of levodopa. Younger patients, in particular, are more likely to show response fluctuations, so other antiparkinsonian drugs should be considered first to delay the introduction of levodopa. After 5 years of treatment with levodopa, 91% of young patients had motor fluctuations and dyskinesias. After 10 years, 100% were so affected.[5]

Patients with mild symptoms may be treated in several ways. Choices include:

- Deferring symptomatic medications until it seems appropriate to start levodopa therapy
- Initiating treatment with a dopamine agonist, an anticholinergic drug, or amantadine
- Introducing an MAO-B inhibitor.

Dosage and administration data for the antiparkinson agents are summarized in **Table 8.1**.

Anticholinergics

Because of the relative sparing of the cholinergic system in PD, coupled with a marked depletion of dopamine, the acetylcholine-dopamine balance in the striatum of PD is tilted in favor of the cholinergic pathways. Not surprisingly, therefore, the symptoms of PD are responsive to anticholinergic agents, which antagonize the cholinergic neurons disinhibited by the loss of dopaminergic neurons.

Anticholinergic agents, the oldest class of drugs used in the treatment of PD, can still be helpful. They are generally thought to be effective for the symptoms of tremor, as rigidity and bradykinesia are not much altered. (However, the response of tremor to anticholinergics as well as to other drugs is highly variable.)

And, in some cases, they may be useful adjuvants to levodopa therapy, particularly in patients with motor fluctuations.

■ **Dosage and Administration**
- Trihexyphenidyl (Artane)
  - Initiate with 1 mg at mealtime
  - Increase 2 mg/day for 3 to 5 days to 6 mg/day tid at mealtimes
- Benztropine (Cogentin)
  - Initiate with 0.5 mg to 1 mg at bedtime
  - Can increase to 4 mg to 6 mg/day bid or qid, if needed
- Procyclidine (Kemadrin)
  - Initiate with 2.5 mg tid after meals
  - Increase to 5 mg/day tid or qid.

8

These drugs have a number of side effects, including:
- Dry mouth
- Narrow-angle glaucoma
- Constipation
- Urinary retention
- Memory impairment
- Confusion/hallucinations.

The anticholinergics should be used with caution, if at all, in the elderly since they have a poor therapeutic index and high toxicity.

Amantadine (Symmetrel)

Patients whose early symptoms do not respond to anticholinergics may benefit from substitution by or addition of amantadine. An antiviral agent found to have an antiparkinsonian effect as well, amantadine's precise mechanism of action remains to be defined. However, it releases dopamine from peripheral neu-

TABLE 8.1 — Antiparkinsonian Agents

Generic (Trade) Name	Recommended Dosage	Comments
Anticholinergics	—	Effective for tremor (variably); use with caution in elderly
Benztropine (Cogentin)	Initiate: 0.5-1 mg/d at bedtime; can increase to 4-6 mg/d in divided doses	
Procyclidine (Kemadrin)	Initiate: 2.5 mg tid after meals; increase to 5 mg tid or qid	—
Trihexyphenidyl (Artane)	Initiate: First day, 1 mg at mealtime; increase 2 mg/d for 3-5 d to 6 mg/d tid at mealtimes	—
Dopamine Agonists	—	Most effective drugs after levodopa; may be used as monotherapy
Bromocriptine (Parlodel)	Initiate: 1/2 of 2.5-mg tablet with meals bid; increase slowly to 5-15 mg/d	—
Pergolide (Permax)	Initiate: 0.05 mg/d for 2 d; increase 0.10 or 0.15 mg/d q third d for 12 d; increase 0.25 mg/d to 3 mg/d tid	New physician warning regarding valvular heart defects, especially with doses over 5 mg/day

Pramipexole (Mirapex)	Initiate: 0.125 mg tid; increase q 5-7 d to 3 mg or 4.5 mg/d tid (See Table 8.2)	Indicated for both monotherapy and as adjunct to levodopa. Advise patient about drowsiness while driving
Ropinirole (Requip)	Initiate: 0.25 mg/d tid; increase weekly by 0.25 mg/d tid to maximum of 24 mg/d tid	Indicated for both monotherapy and as adjunct to levodopa. Advise patient about drowsiness while driving
Levodopa		
Carbidopa/levodopa	Initiate: ½ of 25/100 tablet bid after a meal; increase by ½ tablet/d, q 4-7 d; no maximum	"Gold standard" of parkinsonian therapy. Timing of initiation controversial
Carbidopa/levodopa orally disintegrating tablets (Parcopa)	Same strengths and dosage schedule as conventional carbidopa/levodopa tablets	Can be taken without water
Carbidopa/levodopa controlled-release	Initiate: 25/100 tablet or 50/200 tablet bid; no maximum	Effective for sleep. Just as likely to produce motor fluctuations as regular Sinemet
Cardidopa/levodopa/ entacapone (Stalevo)	In patients already stabilized on carbidopa/ levodopa and entacapone separately, initiate an equivalent dose of carbidopa/levodopa	Available in three strengths, each with a 1:4 ratio of carbidopa to levodopa and 200 mg entacapone

8

Continued

Generic (Trade) Name	Recommended Dosage	Comments
COMT Inhibitors		
Tolcapone (Tasmar)*	100 mg or 200 mg tid (with each dose of levodopa	Adjunct to levodopa. Less restrictive liver monitoring requirements recently approved (see discussion below)
Entacapone (Comtan)	200 mg with each dose of levodopa up to a *maximum of 1600 mg entacapone daily*	Adjunct to levodopa (see also *carbidopa/ levodopa/entacapone* above)
Selective MAO-B Inhibitors		
Selegiline (Eldepryl)	5 mg at breakfast and lunch; 5 mg/d may be effective in some patients	As monotherapy in early PD, delays the need for levodopa. As adjunctive therapy, prolongs the symptomatic benefits of levodopa
Zydis selegiline (Zelapar)	New buccal formulation of selegiline. The tablet should be placed on the tongue in the morning, at least 5 minutes before breakfast. Start at 1.25 mg once daily for 6 weeks, then increase as needed to a maximum of 2.5 mg once daily	Adjunctive use to reduce "off" time in levodopa-treated patients with motor fluctuations

Rasagiline mesylate (Azilect)	The recommended dose is 1 mg once daily as monotherapy in early PD. The recommended starting dose is 0.5 mg once daily as adjunctive therapy in moderate to advanced disease which can be increased to 1.0 mg once daily to improve efficacy	Initial monotherapy in the treatment of early PD and as adjunct to levodopa therapy for moderate to advanced disease
Other		
Amantadine (Symmetrel)	As monotherapy or in combination: 100-400 mg/d	Global improvement of 20% to 40% in 66% of patients; minimal effect on tremor. May improve dyskinesia

Abbreviation: COMT, catechol-*O*-methyltransferase; MAO-B, monoamine oxidase-B; PD, Parkinson's disease.

* Determination of AST and ALT levels required at baseline then periodically (ie, every 2 to 4 weeks) for the first 6 months and periodically thereafter as deemed clinically relevant by the physician.

ronal storage sites of animals who have received infusions of the transmitters, suggesting it might exert a similar action on the residual, intact dopaminergic terminals in the striatum of parkinsonian patients.[6] Among the other reported actions are:

- Release of dopamine from central neurons
- Delay of dopamine uptake by neural cells
- Blockade of NMDA receptors[7]
- Anticholinergic effects.

Although there is a considerable amount of evidence for the effectiveness of amantadine, largely from non-controlled trials, a recent Cochrane Systematic Review of randomized, controlled trials concluded that there is insufficient evidence for its efficacy as monotherapy or adjunctive symptomatic therapy in idiopathic PD.[8] Similarly, the efficacy of adjunctive amantadine for levodopa-induced dyskinesias is supported by many non-controlled trials, but not by evidence from randomized controlled trials.[9] Furthermore, according to a recent report, the antidyskinetic benefit lasts <8 months.[10]

■ **Dosage and Administration**

As monotherapy or in combination with other antiparkinson drugs, it is administered as follows:

- 100 mg bid
- Dose may be increased to 300 to 400 mg if patient tolerates.

Compared with the anticholinergic agents, amantadine is relatively free of side effects, which may include:

- Hallucinations
- Leg edema
- Livedo reticularis (mottled skin) on legs.

MAO-B Inhibitors

■ Selegiline (Eldepryl)

An irreversible inhibitor of MAO-B, an enzyme associated with the outer membrane of mitochondria, selegiline, or L-deprenyl, is indicated as an adjunct to carbidopa/levodopa (see *Carbidopa/Levodopa* below) for patients who exhibit deterioration in response to levodopa.[4] Selegiline has been shown to prolong the symptomatic benefit of levodopa.

Given some evidence that selegiline may have a neuroprotective effect, a large multicenter trial, the Deprenyl and Tocopherol Antioxidant Therapy of Parkinsonism (DATATOP), by the Parkinson Study Group, was designed to determine whether the two agents (deprenyl and tocopherol) could delay the need for levodopa therapy in newly diagnosed patients.[11] The basis for the study, which involved 800 patients, was the finding that inhibition of MAO-B prevented toxin methylphenyltetrahydropyridine (MPTP)-induced parkinsonism in primates.

A symptomatic effect was suggested by improvement of motor scores after the initiation of deprenyl and deterioration of scores on its withdrawal. However, statistically reduced disability compared with placebo was found even among deprenyl patients who initially had no improvement in motor scores, suggesting a neuroprotective effect.

Two extensions of this study followed,[12,13] with the premise that patients who had received selegiline in the prior DATATOP trial should have less advanced disease than the group who had been randomized to placebo. It was expected that these selegiline-treated patients would reach subsequent progression milestones later than placebo-treated patients. This was not the case, however; the frequency of progression sufficient to require levodopa initiation[12] and the frequency of developing levodopa motor complications[13] were similar in the two groups. One more recent report showed that the selegiline group had a statistically significant decreased risk for developing freezing of gait.[14] Despite some strong evidence of selegiline's possible neuroprotective effect, however, it remains to be proven.[15] Furthermore, if the drug does influence disease progression, it seems only to mildly slow the course; progression is not halted.[16]

Selegiline Monotherapy

Once the diagnosis of PD is made, selegiline may be offered for some patients with minor nondisabling symptoms. It serves as a hedge against both of the major issues of controversy:[16]

- The initial DATATOP and more recent study results suggesting selegiline's neuroprotective effects
- The oxidant stress hypothesis, which predicts that levodopa treatment toxicity will be reduced by selegiline inhibition of MAO-B oxidation of dopamine.

Appropriate candidates for selegiline monotherapy are:

- Early-stage patients without disabling symptoms
- Young patients (≤65 years of age).

Higher doses provide no additional therapeutic advantages, and doses >30 mg/day also inhibit monoamine oxidase type A (MAO-A), with the potential for hypertensive crisis ("cheese" effect). However, the cheese effect is not a concern with conventional dosage, thus no dietary modifications are necessary.

According to the DATATOP trials, selegiline monotherapy is typically well tolerated, at least early in Parkinson patients.[11,13] The drug should probably not be prescribed to cognitively impaired patients since it could lead to cognitive decompensation and psychosis.

A recent evidence-based review of pharmacological treatments of PD concluded that there is insufficient evidence to use selegiline monotherapy for the prevention of clinical progression.[17]

Selegiline as Adjunctive Therapy

A recent evidence-based review of pharmacological treatments of PD concluded that there is insufficient evidence for the efficacy of the traditional oral formulation of selegiline as adjunctive therapy to treat or prevent fluctuations. In addition, it is deemed non-efficacious for the prevention of dyskinesias.[17]

In 1995, the United Kingdom's Parkinson's Research group reported increased mortality from selegiline when used with levodopa.[18] This report has been challenged for methodological problems and the results are not consistent with subsequent studies.[19,20] The most recent study, a meta-analysis of 17 randomized trials involving 3,525 patients found no significant difference in mortality between patients on MAO-B inhibitors and control patients.[21]

A recent evidence-based practice parameter published by the American Academy of Neurology states that adjunctive selegiline may be considered to reduce off time (evidence level C).[22]

Dosage and Administration
- 10 mg/day, 5 mg at breakfast and lunch
- 5 mg/day may be effective in some patients.

■ Zydis Selegiline (Zelapar)

This new formulation of selegiline, recently approved by the FDA, dissolves on contact with saliva and is rapidly absorbed through the buccal mucosa, thereby minimizing first-pass metabolism.[23] This results in a high plasma concentration of selegiline and a 3-fold to 10-fold reduction in amphetamine metabolites. By using the zydis formulation, the conventional

10 mg oral dose of selegiline can be reduced 4- to 5-fold. The effectiveness of adjunctive zydis selegiline (1.25 mg to 2.5 mg daily) was demonstrated in a double-blind, randomized, 12-week trial in patients who were levodopa responsive and exhibited dose deterioration with at least 3 hours "off" time/day.[24] As can be seen in **Figure 8.2**, there were significant reductions in daily "off" time at 4 to 6 weeks with the 1.25-mg dose (9.9%; $P = 0.003$), and at 10 to 12 weeks with the 2.5-mg dose (13.2%; $P < 0.001$). The total number of "off" hours was reduced from baseline by 2.2 hours at week 12 (compared with 0.6 hours in the placebo group). In addition, the average number of "dyskinesia-free on" hours increased by 1.8 hours in the zydis selegiline patients. Ondo reported pooled analysis of the results from two identical 12-week phase 3 clinical trials.[25] Intention to treat analysis included 192 patients who received zydis selegiline and

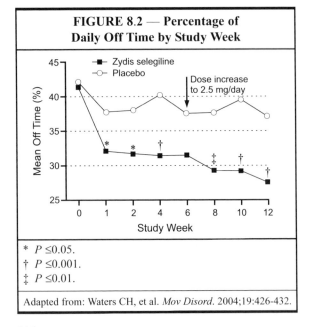

FIGURE 8.2 — Percentage of Daily Off Time by Study Week

* $P \leq 0.05$.
† $P \leq 0.001$.
‡ $P \leq 0.01$.

Adapted from: Waters CH, et al. *Mov Disord*. 2004;19:426-432.

96 who received placebo. The results at 10 and 12 weeks showed a 12.4% reduction in percentage of mean daily "off" time in the active treatment group compared with a 6.9% in the placebo group ($P = 0.004$). These percentage reductions correlated with 4.7 ± 1.9 daily "off" hours in the zydis selegiline group vs 5.7 ± 2.8 daily "off" hours in the placebo group ($P = 0.004$).

Dosage and Administration

The recommended daily dose of zydis selegiline is 2.5 mg/day. Treatment should be initiated with 1.25 mg given once a day for at least 6 weeks. After 6 weeks, the dose may be escalated to 2.5 mg given once a day if a desired benefit has not been achieved and the patient is tolerating zydis selegiline. There is no evidence that doses >2.5 mg/day confer any additional benefit, and they should ordinarily be avoided because of the potential increased risk of adverse events. Zydis selegiline is contraindicated for concomitant use with other selegiline-containing medications, meperidine and certain other analgesics, dextromethorphan, MAO inhibitors, and sympathomimetic amines, including amphetamines and medicines containing vasoconstrictors such as pseudoephedrine, phenylephrine, phenylpropanolamine, and ephedrine. Use with tricyclic or SSRI antidepressants is also not recommended.

Zydis selegiline should be taken in the morning before breakfast and without liquid. The tablet should be placed on the tongue in the morning, at least 5 minutes before breakfast, and allowed to dissolve. The patients should not eat, drink, or rinse the mouth for at least 5 minutes after taking the medicine.

■ Rasagiline (Azilect)

Rasagiline is a second-generation, irreversible, selective MAO-B that has been shown to exhibit neuroprotective properties in cell and animal models via a mechanism other than MAO-B inhibition.[26-28]

Unlike selegiline, rasagiline is not metabolized to amphetamine derivatives. Rasagiline is the only MAO-B inhibitor approved in the United States for use both as initial monotherapy in the treatment of early PD and as an adjunct to levodopa therapy for moderate to advanced disease.

An early, small, 10-week, randomized, placebo-controlled, monotherapy trial in early PD found that rasagiline was safe and well tolerated and improved the UPDRS scores.[29] The subsequent 26-week, parallel-group, randomized, double-blind, placebo-controlled TVP-1012 in Early Monotherapy for Parkinson's Disease Outpatients (TEMPO) study randomized 404 patients with early PD not requiring dopaminergic therapy to receive rasagiline 1 mg, 2 mg, or placebo.[30] The primary end point was the change in the total UPDRS score between baseline and 26 weeks. Unlike the DATATOP study (see above), the TEMPO study was not designed or powered to assess time to levodopa or time to additional dopaminergic therapy as end points. As shown in **Figure 8.3**, both dosages of rasagiline were significantly more effective than placebo (change from baseline, 0.1 and 0.7 with the 1-mg and 2-mg dose, respectively, vs 3.9 with placebo; $P = 0.0001$ for both). Of the 138 patients in the placebo group, 23 (16.7%) reached the secondary end point of requiring levodopa therapy compared with 15 (11.2%) of 134 patients and 22 (16.7%) of 132 patients in the 1-mg and 2-mg rasagiline groups, respectively. Results from the 328 patients who completed 6 months without additional therapy were similar to those shown from all completing patients. Both rasagiline groups showed significant improvements in PD quality of life (PDQUALIF) scores compared with the placebo group. There were no meaningful differences in the frequency of adverse events or premature discontinuations among the three treatment groups.

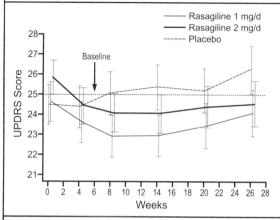

FIGURE 8.3 — Total Unadjusted Unified Parkinson's Disease Rating Scale Score by Visit for Each Treatment Group

Abbreviations: SE, standard error; UPDRS, Unified Parkinson's Disease Rating Scale.

Error bars indicate ± 1 SE.

Adapted from: Parkinson Study Group. *Arch Neurol.* 2002;59: 1937-1943.

In an extension phase of the TEMPO trial, patients originally randomized to rasagiline continued on their same dose, while those previously randomized to placebo received rasagiline 2 mg per day.[31] The 1-year data were analyzed as a randomized, delayed-start clinical trial. The objective was to assess whether earlier initiation of rasagiline resulted in better functional status at 1 year. Patients treated with rasagiline 2 and 1 mg per day for 12 months demonstrated a significantly less functional decline that those in whom treatment was delayed for 6 months. According to the investigators, the randomized, delayed-start analysis suggests that the effects of rasagiline on progression cannot be fully explained by its symptomatic effect and may be due to a disease-modifying effect.

Two large randomized, controlled trials evaluated rasagiline as adjunctive therapy in patients with levodopa motor complications. The Parkinson's Rasagiline: Efficacy and Safety in the Treatment of "Off" (PRESTO) trial was a 26-week trial in 472 levodopa-treated patients with at least 2½ hours of daily "off" time despite optimized treatment with other anti-PD medications.[32] Patients were randomized to receive rasagiline 0.5 or 1 mg/day or placebo. The levodopa dosage could be decreased during the first 6 weeks at the discretion of the investigator but was held constant for the last 20 weeks of the study. The primary end point was change from baseline in mean total daily off time measured by patient diaries. During the treatment period, the mean adjusted total daily off time decreased from baseline by 1.85 hours (29%; $P = 0.02$ vs placebo) in the 0.5-mg rasagiline group, 1.41 hours (23%; $P < 0.001$ in the 1.0-mg rasagiline group, and 0.91 hour in the placebo group) (**Figure 8.4**). Several prespecified secondary end points were also assessed. Compared with placebo, the clinical global impression, UPDRS ADL score during off time, and the UPDRS motor score during on time improved significantly during treatment with either dose of rasagiline. Both doses of rasagiline were well tolerated. None of the serious adverse events were significantly more common in patients receiving rasagiline compared with placebo.

A second, 18-week, adjunctive study, the Lasting Effect in Adjunct Therapy With Rasagiline Given Once Daily (LARGO) trial, compared treatment with rasagiline 1 mg per day with entacapone 200 mg tid (ie, with each levodopa dose) and placebo in 687 levodopa-treated patients with motor fluctuations.[33] The primary outcome was change from baseline in total daily "off" time. Other measures included the clinical global improvement (CGI) score and UPDRS scores. Both

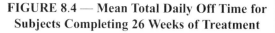

FIGURE 8.4 — Mean Total Daily Off Time for Subjects Completing 26 Weeks of Treatment

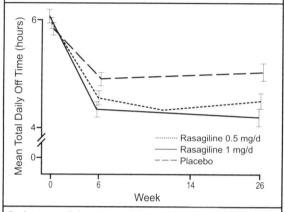

.... Rasagiline 0.5 mg/d
——— Rasagiline 1 mg/d
– – – Placebo

Patients receiving 0.5 or 1.0 mg/day of rasagiline had a greater reduction in mean total daily off time compared with patients receiving placebo.

Adapted from: Parkinson Study Group. *Arch Neurol.* 2005;62: 241-248.

rasagiline (–1.18 hr) and entacapone (–1.2 hr) significantly reduced mean daily off time as compared with placebo (–0.4 hr) and increased daily on time without troublesome dyskinesias (**Figure 8.5**). Adjunctive treatment with rasagiline and entacapone also resulted in significant improvements in CGI scores and improvements in UPDRS scores for ADL during off time, and motor function during on time. While the incidence of postural hypotension was greater with rasagiline than with placebo, other side effects with rasagiline were similar to those with placebo.

A recent evidence-based practice parameter published by the American Academy of Neurology states that adjunctive rasagiline should be offered to reduce off time (evidence level A).[22]

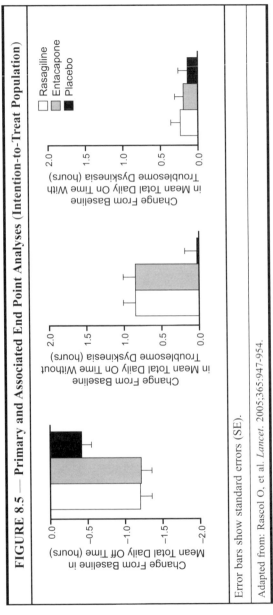

FIGURE 8.5 — Primary and Associated End Point Analyses (Intention-to-Treat Population)

Error bars show standard errors (SE).

Adapted from: Rascol O, et al. *Lancet*. 2005;365:947-954.

Dosage and Administration

The recommended dose for rasagiline monotherapy in early Parkinson's disease is 1 mg daily. The recommended starting dose of rasagiline as adjunctive therapy in patients with moderate to advanced disease is 0.5 mg daily and may be increased to 1.0 mg for greater efficacy. If there is an increase in dyskinesias during adjunct use of rasagiline with levodopa, the dose of levodopa should be reduced.

Doses should not exceed 0.5 mg/day in patients with mild hepatic impairment and those receiving concomitant treatment with ciprofloxacin and other CYP1A2 inhibitors. Patients with moderate or severe decreases in liver function should not receive rasagiline. Rasagiline is contraindicated for concomitant use with meperidine and certain other analgesics, dextromethorphan, MAO inhibitors, and sympathomimetic amines, including amphetamines and medicines containing vasoconstrictors such as pseudoephedrine, phenylephrine, phenylpropanolamine, and ephedrine. Patients should be instructed about food containing high amounts of tyramine and told to avoid those while taking rasagiline. It is necessary to maintain this dietary tyramine restriction for 2 weeks following the discontinuation of rasagiline.

Dopamine Agonists

Unlike levodopa, dopamine agonist agents do not require conversion and storage because they bypass the failing nigrostriatal pathway to directly stimulate receptors in the normal striatum. They are the most effective class of drugs for PD after levodopa. In early disease, they may be equally as beneficial as levodopa and provide an effective treatment strategy, delaying the need for levodopa. Four dopamine agonists are currently available in the United States:

- Bromocriptine (Parlodel)

- Pergolide (Permax)
- Pramipexole (Mirapex)
- Ropinirole (Requip).

Cabergoline (Casbar) is available elsewhere.

Dopamine agonists have longer half-lives than levodopa (**Table 8.2**). There is some evidence that dopamine agonists are associated with less risk of the development of dyskinesia than levodopa. There is recent compelling evidence with the dopamine agonists that levodopa can be delayed for a number of years. Therefore, I recommend the use of these compounds prior to levodopa initiation early in the disease to avoid or delay the production of dyskinesia, especially in patients who are young.[3]

The basis for the development of dyskinesia appears to depend on disease severity and the half-life of the dopaminergic agent. Patients who have mild disease do not develop dyskinesia with either levodopa or dopamine agonists, presumably because they still have enough dopamine terminals to regulate dopamine release and provide postsynaptic dopamine receptors with relatively physiologic dopaminergic stimulation. In more advanced disease, there are not enough

TABLE 8.2 — Half-Life of Dopamine Agents		
Trade Name	**Generic Name**	**Half-Life**
Sinemet	Carbidopa/levodopa	1-1.5 h
Parlodel	Bromocriptine	12-15 h
Permax	Pergolide	7-16 h
Requip	Ropinirole	6-8 h
Mirapex	Pramipexole	8-12 h
Casbar	Cabergoline	>24 h
Olanow W, et al. *Trends Neurosci.* 2000;23(10 suppl):S117-S126.		

dopamine terminals to regulate dopamine release, resulting in fluctuations in striatal levodopa. The resulting exposure of striatal receptors to alternating high and low concentrations of dopamine seems to induce the postsynaptic changes that lead to the development of dyskinesia and motor complications. Dopamine agonists that act directly on the dopamine receptor have the potential to provide longer, more physiologic stimulation of receptors and prevent development of such changes. Unlike levodopa, with its brief half-life of 60 to 90 minutes, dopamine agonists have a lesser propensity to produce dyskinesias.

Initial monotherapy with dopamine agonists may be more useful in younger patients. They are more prone to the early development of levodopa-related clinical fluctuations and will have to be treated for a longer time than those who are older at the time of onset.

The question of whether early combination therapy with lower-dose levodopa and a dopamine agonist will delay disability has no definitive answer. The use of the dopamine agonists to prolong the symptomatic benefit of levodopa in patients with advanced, fluctuating disease is discussed in Chapter 9, *Complications of Parkinson's Disease and Its Therapy.*

■ **Bromocriptine (Parlodel)**

An ergot alkaloid with potent D_2 agonist effects, bromocriptine is approved as adjunctive therapy with carbidopa/levodopa for patients who develop tolerance to levodopa and experience end-of-dose failure.[6]

Dosage and Administration
- Initial dose, 1/2 of a 2.5-mg tablet bid with meals
- Increase slowly
- Therapeutic dose is usually 5 mg to 30 mg/day.

The addition of bromocriptine may permit reduction in the maintenance dose of levodopa.

The most common side effects of bromocriptine are:

- Nausea
- Dyskinesia
- Hallucinations
- Confusion
- Postural hypotension.

A variety of bromocriptine dosage regimens have been used as monotherapy in the treatment of early or mild PD. Studies have shown significantly more adverse reactions in bromocriptine-treated than in carbidopa/levodopa-treated patients.

■ **Pergolide (Permax)**

Also an ergot derivative, pergolide stimulates both D_1 and D_2 dopamine receptors. Like bromocriptine, it is indicated as adjunctive treatment with carbidopa/levodopa. A recent evidence-based practice parameter published by the American Academy of Neurology states that adjunctive pergolide should be considered to reduce off time (evidence level B).[22]

Pergolide has only infrequently been studied in the treatment of early PD. One double-blind, 3-year study (the PELMOPET study) was conducted in 294 patients who were randomized either to levodopa or pergolide.[34] The time to onset of motor complications was significantly longer with pergolide than with levodopa. Also, the motor complications in this group were less severe. The efficacy of levodopa, however, was superior to that of pergolide. The PET component of this study did not show any difference in progression of the disease between the two groups. Adverse events leading to discontinuation was higher for pergolide (17.6%) than levodopa (9.6%).

Dosage and Administration
- Initiate with 0.05 mg/day for first 2 days
- Increase gradually by 0.10 or 0.15 mg/day every third day over next 12 days
- Increase by 0.25 mg/day every third day to optimal dose
- Therapeutic dose range is 0.75 mg to 6 mg/day in divided doses tid.

Such gradual titration is important, given the approximately 10% of patients in clinical trials who experienced symptomatic, orthostatic, and/or sustained hypotension.

The other most commonly seen side effects of pergolide are:
- Dyskinesia
- Hallucinations
- Somnolence
- Insomnia
- Nausea
- Constipation
- Diarrhea
- Dyspepsia.

Because of new serious warnings about pergolide and valvular heart disease,[35] it should rarely be considered except in patients who do not tolerate other dopamine agonists. Patients remaining on pergolide should have annual echocardiograms.

■ Cabergoline (Casbar)
This long-acting ergot-derived dopamine agonist has been studied in early and advanced Parkinson's disease.[36] Cabergoline is not available in the United States, but it can be used in other countries. In a multicenter randomized double-blind 3- to 5-year trial, cabergoline was used alone or in combination with levodopa in early PD. Patients were evaluated for the

development of motor complications. The study medication was titrated over 24 weeks and when the dose was optimized, it was maintained. The end point was the development of motor complications confirmed at two consecutive visits. Open-label levodopa was added in both arms of the study if benefit fell below 30% of baseline. Both treatments improved motor disability. Cabergoline resulted in fewer motor complications than occurred in levodopa-treated patients. Side effects were somewhat greater with cabergoline than with levodopa.

There also has been some concern that cabergoline, like pergolide, may be associated with valvular heart disease.[37] Patients remaining on cabergoline should have annual echocardiograms.

■ Pramipexole (Mirapex)

Pramipexole is a non-ergot benzothiazole derivative. It is a potent dopamine benzothiazole agonist that binds to the D_3 receptor subtype of the D_2 receptor class.[38] The indication for pramipexole is somewhat broader than that for the ergot derivatives bromocriptine and pergolide for the treatment of the signs and symptoms of PD.

Pramipexole as Monotherapy

A 24-week multicenter, randomized, double-blind trial involved 335 early-stage patients who were not receiving levodopa.[39] In each case, study medication was titrated to the patient's maximally well-tolerated dose for up to 7 weeks before the 6-month follow-up. Results included:

- Pramipexole significantly reduced the severity of PD as measured by decreases in parts II (activities of daily living) and III (motor signs) of the Unified Parkinson's Disease Rating Scale (UPDRS)

- Only nausea, constipation, and insomnia had a 10% higher incidence rate in pramipexole patients compared with those who received placebo
- No clinically significant changes were noted in blood pressure or pulse rate.

A 10-week randomized dose-ranging (1.5 to 6.0 mg/day) trial, which involved 264 patients who had not received levodopa, also found pramipexole to be safe and effective as short-term monotherapy.[40] Findings were:
- A 20% improvement in total UPDRS scores, largely motor benefits, similar for all dosages
- Evidence that treatment effects were more pronounced in subjects with worse UPDRS scores at baseline
- Somnolence was reported with greater frequency in the pramipexole group.

Pramipexole was also compared with levodopa in another multicenter randomized, parallel group double-blind study conducted by the Parkinson Study Group.[41] In this study, 301 patients were randomized to pramipexole (0.5 mg tid) or carbidopa/levodopa (25/100 mg tid). The dose could be escalated for the first 10 weeks. Open-label levodopa was permitted for emerging disability during the study. There were three outcome measures:
- Time to first occurrence of any of three dopaminergic complications (wearing off, dyskinesias, or on-off fluctuations)
- Changes in scores on the UPDRS assessed baseline and follow-up
- Single photon emission computed tomography (SPECT) measured dopamine uptake in a subgroup of 82 subjects (designed to assess neuroprotection).

After 2 years, pramipexole was associated with significantly less dyskinesia, wearing off, and motor fluctuations (28%) than levodopa (51%). The levodopa group showed a significant improvement in the total UPDRS scores compared with the pramipexole group when the scores at 23.5 months were compared with baseline. Somnolence was more common in the pramipexole group (32.4% vs 17.3%). There was no difference between the two groups in the SPECT study. A quality-of-life analysis showed greater improvement in the levodopa group. Several patients experienced sudden sleepiness (although one was in the levodopa group).

The above study was extended to a minimum of 4 years.[42] The results are shown in **Figure 8.6**. Compared with levodopa, initial treatment with pramipexole resulted in a significant reduction in the risk of developing dyskinesias (24.5% vs 54%, $P < 0.001$) and wearing off (47% vs 62.7%, $P = 0.02$). However, compared with pramipexole, initial treatment with levodopa resulted in a significant reduction in the risk of freezing (25.3% vs 37.1%, $P = 0.01$). By 48 months, the occurrence of disabling dyskinesias was uncommon and did not differ significantly between treatments. At 48 months, the mean improvement over the baseline total UPDRS score was significantly greater ($P = 0.003$) in the levodopa group. There was no between-group difference in the mean changes in quality-of-life scores. The incidence of somnolence and edema was greater in the pramipexole group.

Pramipexole as Adjunctive Therapy

A US study of pramipexole as adjunct therapy was conducted in two parts: a 32-week, double-blind, placebo-controlled parallel-group study, followed by an open-label extension trial.[43] Of 360 patients with advanced disease and "wearing-off" phenomenon, 181 were randomized to pramipexole (0.375 mg to 4.5 mg/

day, increased daily to maximal tolerated or stable improvement), and 179 to placebo.

The primary end points were change from baseline to final maintenance visit of the average of the "on" and "off" ratings for:
- UPDRS part II (activities of daily living)
- UPDRS part III (parkinsonian motor signs).

A number of secondary end points included changes from baseline to final visit in Schwab and England Disability Scale, Hoehn and Yahr stage, and patient diaries.

Patients were followed for 6 months. Compared with placebo, pramipexole at a maximal daily dosage of 4.5 mg:
- Improved activities of daily living as determined by UPDRS part II, assessed in the "on" and "off" periods and averaged
- Improved motor function as determined by UPDRS part III motor evaluation, assessed in the "on" period
- An overall statistically significant decrease in the severity of the "off" periods (**Figure 8**.7)
- A 27% reduction in the dosage of levodopa.

The magnitude of improvement in activities of daily living (21%), motor evaluation (25%), and time in the "off" period (31%) compared favorably with that of other dopamine agonists. Central nervous system adverse events were also similar. Gastrointestinal and cardiovascular side effects were less frequent.

The open-label extension of this trial revealed good tolerability of pramipexole over 4 years' duration.[44]

Another randomized, double-blind, placebo-controlled study of pramipexole as adjunctive therapy was conducted in 354 patients with advanced PD and "end of dose" motor fluctuations who were receiving stable,

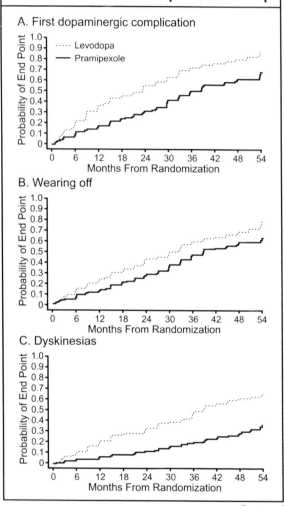

FIGURE 8.6 — Risk of Developing
Dopaminergic Complications Over 4 Years:
Initial Treatment With Pramipexole vs Levodopa

A. First dopaminergic complication

B. Wearing off

C. Dyskinesias

Continued

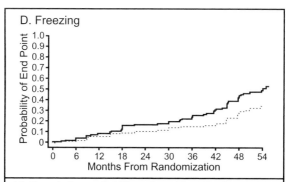

D. Freezing

(A) Cumulative probability of reaching the first dopaminergic complicaton (defined as first occurrence of wearing off, dyskinesias, or on-off fluctuations); (B) wearing off; (C) dyskinesias; and (D) freezing.

Holloway RG, et al. *Arch Neurol*. 2004;61:1044-1053.

8

individually adjusted levodopa.[45] The trial included an ascending-dose phase of up to 7 weeks and a maintenance phase of up to 24 weeks. Pramipexole dihydrochloride or matching placebo was administered tid as an adjunct to levodopa in seven dosages from 0.375 to 4.5 mg per day (corresponding to pramipexole 0.26 to 3.15 mg per day). The double-blind phase was followed by an open-label extension trial with a maximum duration of 57 months.

During the double-blind phase, pramipexole improved UPDRS sum scores of parts II and III by 30% and decreased "off" time by approximately 2.5 hours per day. Compared with placebo, the differences became significant at a daily dose of 0.75 mg per day of pramipexole. A subsequent *post hoc* analysis was performed to assess the effect of pramipexole on resting tremor and depression. Compared with placebo, patients with pronounced resting tremor at enrollment derived a clear benefit with pramipexole. Pramipexole also improved the subitems motivation/initiative and

FIGURE 8.7 — "Off" Periods Associated With Pramipexole and Placebo

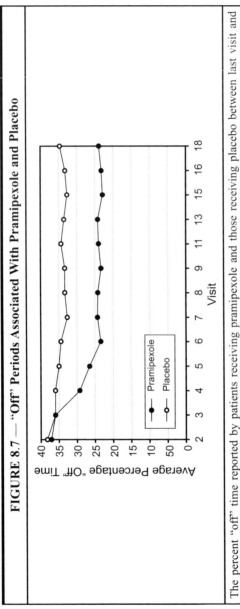

The percent "off" time reported by patients receiving pramipexole and those receiving placebo between last visit and baseline shows a statistically significant decrease in favor of pramipexole.

Adapted from: Lieberman A, et al. *Neurology.* 1997;49:162-168.

depression in the subpopulation of patients who exhibited increased UPDRS Scale I scores at enrollment.

Although there was a moderate decrease in clinical improvement during the long-term open-label phase, this was anticipated taking into account the usual disease progression over a >4-year period in some patients

During the open-label study, the most frequent drug-related adverse events included asymptomatic and symptomatic orthostatic hypotension, dyskinesia, visual hallucinations, and nausea. During the open-label phase, the rate of adverse events did not increase with time but remained constant. In the double-blind study, somnolence was spontaneously reported by three patients in the pramipexole group versus four in the placebo group. In the open-label study, somnolence was observed in seven patients. No motor vehicle accidents or events of falling asleep at the wheel were recorded.

Wong and associates evaluated the efficacy and safety of pramipexole in levodopa-naïve (n = 43) and levodopa-treated (n = 104) patients with early or advanced PD in a 15-week (7-week dose-escalation and 8 weeks maintenance), randomized, double-blind, placebo-controlled trial.[46] Overall, pramipexole was significantly more effective than placebo. At week 15, UPDRS Part II + III scores (the primary end point) improved by 12.14 points on pramipexole and 2.45 on placebo (P <0.001). Regardless of levodopa use, the mean UPDRS scores showed a consistently greater improvement in patients receiving pramipexole than in those receiving placebo. In addition, the mean number of off hours in levodopa-treated patients decreased from baseline 7.07 to 6.15 hours/day at end point in pramipexole patient whereas mean off hours increased from baseline 5.59 to 6.87 in placebo-treated patients.

Another recent prospective, 11-week, randomized, placebo-controlled trial evaluated the effectiveness of adjunctive pramipexole in 84 PD patients with "drug-resistant" tremor who were receiving stable, optimized antiparkinsonian medications.[47] The primary end point was the absolute change in the sum of tremor items in the UPDRS. At study end point, pramipexole was significantly ($P < 0.0001$) superior to placebo with a difference between treatment groups in the mean absolute change in tremor score of –4.4, corresponding to a mean relative change of –34.7%.

A recent evidence-based practice parameter published by the American Academy of Neurology states that adjunctive pramipexole should be considered to reduce off time (evidence level B).[22]

Dosage and Administration

Pramipexole should be titrated gradually to achieve a maximum therapeutic effect balanced against the principal side effects of dyskinesia, hallucinations, somnolence, and dry mouth. For initial treatment:

- Increase gradually from a starting dose of 0.125 mg/day tid
- Should not be increased more frequently than every 5 to 7 days.

A suggested ascending dosage schedule, which was used in clinical studies, is shown in **Table 8**.**3**. There are other dosing recommendations for patients with renal impairment that involve reducing the frequency and thus the total maximum daily dose.

There is strong evidence that pramipexole is an excellent medication for early PD. Its role in more advanced disease seems to be similar to that seen with other dopamine agonists.

Adverse experiences with pramipexole were found to be similar to those of other dopamine agonists, although symptomatic orthostatic hypotension was uncommon. A recent report documents a rare but serious occurrence of sudden sleep attacks while driving

136

TABLE 8.3 — Ascending Dosage Schedule for Pramipexole (Mirapex)		
Week	**Dosage (mg)**	**Total Daily Dose (mg)**
1	0.125 tid	0.375
2	0.25 tid	0.75
3	0.5 tid	1.5
4	0.75 tid	2.25
5	1.0 tid	3.0
6	1.25 tid	3.75
7	1.5 tid	4.5

that resulted in accidents.[48] Patients may have no warning prior to these attacks. Eight patients were described; seven who were receiving pramipexole and one receiving ropinirole. Patients should be advised of this potential side effect (see Chapter 9, *Complications of Parkinson's Disease and Its Therapy*, Sleep Disorders section).

■ Ropinirole (Requip)

Ropinirole has a novel, nonergoline structure closely similar to that of dopamine.[49] This chemical structure has the potential to maintain a structure-activity relationship similar to that of dopamine and other effective dopamine agonists without producing ergot-related adverse effects. Ropinirole has been shown to exert a presynaptic effect via stimulation of dopamine D_2 and D_3 receptors, binding with a higher affinity to D_3 receptors.

Ropinirole as Monotherapy

Ropinirole has been assessed as monotherapy in early disease in three double-blind, randomized, controlled multicenter trials[50]:

- A 6-month placebo-controlled trial involving 241 patients (with a 6-month extension)[51]
- A 5-year levodopa-controlled study of 268 patients[52]
- A 3-year bromocriptine-controlled trial (prospectively stratified for selegiline use) of 335 patients.[53]

Patients enrolled in these studies had early PD, had not been treated with levodopa (or treated for no more than 6 weeks) and, in the investigators' opinion, were in need of dopaminergic therapy. Ropinirole and comparator were titrated according to patient response, and the principal measure of efficacy was the UPDRS.

To summarize the efficacy of ropinirole as monotherapy during the first 6 months of treatment of early PD:

- Patients on ropinirole showed statistically significant improvement in the UPDRS motor scores (24% reduction) compared with placebo (3% worsening).
- Ropinirole was as effective as levodopa in early disease.
- Ropinirole was significantly superior to bromocriptine in patients not receiving selegiline measured by motor scores (**Figure 8.8**) and activities of daily living scores.

In a 6-month extension study of the first (241 patients) of the three trials, 147 of the patients were continued on double-blind medication without interruption.[54] Of those receiving ropinirole, 44% remained on ropinirole alone without addition of levodopa compared with 22.4% of placebo patients. The ropinirole group also experienced a 30% reduction in UPDRS motor score as well as significant improvement on the clinical global impression (CGI) scale. Ropinirole continued to be well tolerated, with only three patients

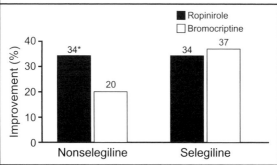

FIGURE 8.8 — Ropinirole and Bromocriptine as Monotherapy: Comparative Improvement in UPDRS Motor Score

* Significantly different from bromocriptine.

On the Unified Parkinson's Disease Rating Scale (UPDRS) motor score, ropinirole alone, without selegiline, was significantly superior to bromocriptine alone in patients with early Parkinson's disease who had not been treated with levodopa (or treated no more than 6 weeks).

Adapted from: Korczyn AD, et al. *Neurology*. 1999;53:364-370.

withdrawing because of adverse experiences. All three clinical trials have been designed to test the efficacy of ropinirole efficacy as early therapy and to determine its ability to replace or significantly delay the need for levodopa.

In a prospective, randomized double-blind study, ropinirole was compared with levodopa for safety and efficacy in early disease.[52] Patients were randomly assigned to a drug (ropinirole or levodopa in a 2:1 ratio). Levodopa supplement was allowed for need. The primary outcome measure was dyskinesia (**Figure 8.9**). One hundred seventy-nine patients were randomly assigned to ropinirole and 89 to levodopa. The patient demographics of the two groups were similar. Twenty-six of the 179 patients assigned to ropinirole had some

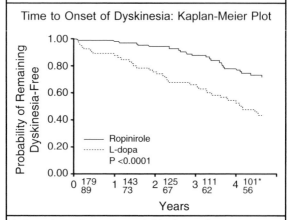

FIGURE 8.9 — Dyskinesias: All Patients, Regardless of Levodopa Supplementation

Time to Onset of Dyskinesia: Kaplan-Meier Plot

Probability of Remaining Dyskinesia-Free

— Ropinirole
······· L-dopa
P <0.0001

Years

	0	1	2	3	4
	179	143	125	111	101*
	89	73	67	62	56

* Low denominator beyond this time point.

The hazard ratio for remaining free of dyskinesias in the ropinirole group as compared with the levodopa group was 2.82 (95% confidence interval, 1.78 to 4.44).

Rascol O, et al. *N Engl J Med.* 2000;342:1484-1491.

exposure to levodopa (<6 weeks) and seven of the 89 in the levodopa group had been exposed to levodopa. The baseline UPDRS scores were identical. About half of the patients in each group completed the 5-year trial. At 5 years, cumulative dyskinesia was 45% in the levodopa group and 20% in the ropinirole group. Before addition of supplementary levodopa, 5% of the ropinirole group and 36% of the levodopa group developed dyskinesia. The levodopa group had significantly better motor scores than those on ropinirole (**Figure 8.10**). There were more hallucinations in the ropinirole group (17%) versus the levodopa group (6%). In a substudy, Korczyn and associates determined that the older patients (>70 years of age) were less likely to tolerate either ropinirole or levodopa than

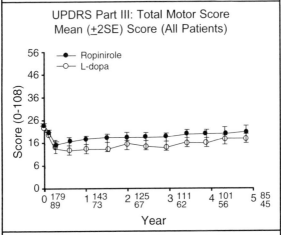

FIGURE 8.10 — Efficacy Assessed by Motor Score

UPDRS Part III: Total Motor Score
Mean (±2SE) Score (All Patients)

Abbreviation: UPDRS, Unified Parkinson's Disease Rating Scale.

The range of possible scores is 0 to 108. Higher scores indicate more severe disability and more severe dysfunction. I bars indicate ± 2 SE.

Rascol O, et al. *N Engl J Med.* 2000;342:1484-1491.

their younger counterparts. There were more hallucinations in the ropinirole group than the levodopa group in the over-70 subset.[55]

The conclusions of these recent monotherapy studies are clear. Dopamine agonists, such as ropinirole, can be used safely and effectively in early PD. There is a substantially reduced risk of dyskinesia during this period of treatment with dopamine agonists.

Ropinirole as Adjunctive Therapy

As an adjunct to levodopa in later-stage patients not adequately controlled with levodopa, ropinirole has been evaluated in four controlled clinical studies.[48]

- A 3-month placebo-controlled trial in 46 patients experiencing mild-to-moderate fluctuations[56]
- A placebo-controlled study of 68 patients with motor fluctuations[50]
- A 6-month, placebo-controlled study of 148 patients not optimally controlled by levodopa[57]
- A 6-month study comparing ropinirole and bromocriptine in 555 patients.[50]

Results of these studies show that when ropinirole is used as an adjunct to levodopa in patients with advanced PD and motor fluctuations:[50]

- Ropinirole reduces awake time spent "off" by an average of 2 to 3 hours when levodopa is not reduced.
- The addition of ropinirole to levodopa allows an average reduction in daily levodopa dose of 20% once a therapeutic dose of the agonist is reached.
- Ropinirole is superior to placebo in generating significant improvement in patients with motor fluctuations.

A recent evidence-based practice parameter published by the American Academy of Neurology states that adjunctive ropinirole should be considered to reduce off time (evidence level B).[22]

Results comparing ropinirole and bromocriptine as adjunctive treatment are unclear.

In monotherapy studies, adverse events with ropinirole are mostly in the range of what is expected of a dopamine agonist. Nausea was the most common but was generally well-tolerated and disappeared over time. (Domperidone, where available, may reduce the nausea.) In adjunct trials, nausea occurred at a much lower rate.

Dizziness, postural hypotension, and syncope were also observed in PD patients and were seen in the ropinirole group as well as in the active comparator groups.

Somnolence occurred in some patients. The incidence of psychiatric episodes was low in the early short-term therapy studies, with no clear differences between confusion and hallucinations with levodopa or bromocriptine.

Dosage and Administration

Whether ropinirole is to be used as monotherapy or as an adjunct to levodopa:

- Initiate therapy with 0.25 mg tid
- Increase in weekly increments (**Table 8**.4)
- Patients may feel benefit by week 4 (1.0 mg tid)
- Dosage should be increased weekly for benefit to a maximum of 8 mg tid
- The titration schedule may be slower, but faster increases are not recommended.

In patients with moderate renal impairment (creatinine clearance, 30 mL to 50 mL/min), no dosage adjustment of ropinirole is necessary. Its use in severe renal impairment has not been studied.

TABLE 8.4 — Ascending Dosage Schedule for Ropinirole (Requip)		
Week	**Dosage (mg)**	**Total Daily Dose (mg)**
1	0.25 tid	0.75 mg
2	0.5 mg tid	1.5 mg
3	0.75 mg tid	2.25 mg
4	1.0 mg tid	3.0 mg
Dosages >24 mg/day have not been tested in clinical trials.		

Thus there is strong evidence that ropinirole is an excellent medicine in early PD. It may substitute for levodopa for several years. As adjunct to levodopa in later disease, it is beneficial in ameliorating the wearing-off phenomenon.

■ **Switching Dopamine Agonists**

There are several dopamine agonists available for use. There has been limited experience with conversion tables and procedures for switching from one dopamine agonist to another. In a recent report by Goetz and associates,[58] patients were switched either suddenly (the next day) or by slow titration (up to 8 weeks). Both groups had a therapeutic response to the new agonist, but the slow-switch group suffered more. It took longer to reach therapeutic levels and two patients were hospitalized with fractures due to falls. Thus the sudden switchover is recommended, whether this is in a patient using a dopamine agonist alone or as an adjunct to levodopa. The conversion factors for the dopamine agonists are shown in **Table 8**.5.

COMT Inhibitors

Although the addition of carbidopa to levodopa increases the amount of the drug available to cross the

TABLE 8.5 — Conversion Factors for the Dopamine Agonists	
Agonist	**Ratio**
Pergolide	1
Pramipexole	1
Ropinirole	4
Bromocriptine	20
Fahn S. 11th Annual Course. A Comprehensive Review of Movement Disorders for the Clinical Practitioner. Aspen, Colo; August 3-6, 2001.	

144

blood-brain barrier, most levodopa is then metabolized in the gut and liver (first-pass metabolism) by COMT to an inactive metabolite, 3-O-methyldopa (3-OMD). The COMT inhibitory agents, tolcapone and entacapone, prevent this breakdown, thus prolonging the half-life of levodopa and increasing its transport into the brain to raise dopamine levels.

■ Tolcapone (Tasmar)

A potent inhibitor of COMT, tolcapone has been investigated as adjunctive therapy with carbidopa/levodopa for both early and mild PD and for advanced disease, complicated by levodopa-related motor fluctuations.[59,60] Treatment with tolcapone resulted in a clinically significant reduction of "off" time, an increase in "on" time, and a reduction in the requirement for levodopa. These results where shown in three multicenter, randomized, controlled trials. Two 3-month trials randomized patients with documented episodes of "wearing off" phenomena despite optimal levodopa therapy to receive placebo, tolcapone 100 mg tid, or tolcapone 200 mg tid.

One of these studies randomized 202 patients in 11 centers in the United States and Canada.[61] After 3 months, patients treated with 200 mg tolcapone, daily "off" time was reduced from baseline by 3.25 hours compared with 1.4 hours with placebo (P <0.01). In addition, the mean daily dosage of levodopa was significantly (P <0.001) reduced with both daily dosages of tolcapone (–116 mg with 100 mg tid; –207 mg with 200 mg tid). The second study enrolled 177 patients from 24 centers in Europe.[62] After 3 months, "off" time decreased significantly from baseline with both tolcapone100 mg tid (–31.5%; P <0.05 vs placebo) and 200 mg tid (–26.2%; P <0.01 vs placebo). Compared with placebo, "on" time increased from baseline with both tolcapone 100 mg tid (21.3%; P <0.01) and 200 mg tid (20.6%; P <0.01). Both doses of tolcapone also significantly decreased the mean total daily levodopa dose by ~17%.

The third double-blind, placebo-controlled trial evaluated the long-term effect of adjunctive tolcapone (100 mg and 200 mg tid) on activities of daily living (UPDRS subscale II) and motor function (UPDRS subscale III) in 298 patients on stable doses of levodopa who were not experiencing "wearing-off" phenomena.[60] Both doses of tolcapone produced significant reductions in the UPDRS subscale II (P <0.001 vs placebo) and subscale III scores (P <0.018). The mean total daily dose of levodopa decrease from baseline while it increased in the placebo group (P <0.001 both tolcapone doses vs placebo).

A recent evidence-based practice parameter published by the American Academy of Neurology states that adjunctive tolcapone should be considered to reduce off time (evidence level B).[22]

Shortly after release of tolcapone in late 1997 in Europe and in March 1998 in the United States, four cases of serious hepatotoxicity were reported, three resulting in death. As a result, a black-box warning was added to the package insert for tolcapone in the United States in November 1998. An intensive liver-monitoring program was also mandated. The major features of the revised US prescribing information at that time were:

- An informed consent must be obtained.
- This drug was indicated in those patients who experience motor fluctuation that is not responding to or who are not candidates for other adjunctive therapies.
- This drug should be withdrawn if no benefit is seen in 3 weeks.
- It should not be used with any evidence of liver disease.
- Liver monitoring is required as follows:
  – Year 1, every 2 weeks

- 12 to 18 months, every 4 weeks
- >18 months, every 2 months.
- If a single SGPT/ALT or SGOT/AST level exceeds normal or if signs and symptoms of hepatic failure are seen, the drug should be stopped.

Since the introduction of these restrictive monitoring requirements in November 1998, approximately 80,000 patients have taken tolcapone. A recent review of data from patients who had taken tolcapone found that between February 1997 and May 1999, 156 cases of hepatic-related adverse events were reported, while between June 1999 and August 2004, 67 patients had developed hepatic-related adverse events with six cases of acute hepatitis and one case of severe hepatobiliarly dysfunction.[63] Many of the reported cases involved patients who were taking other medications also associated with the potential development of adverse events.

In Feburary 2006, after a review of >40,000 patient-years of tolcapone prescription data and laboratory data from >3400 tolcapone-treated patients who participated in clinical trials, the FDA approved less restrictive labeling for tolcapone. The new monitoring guidelines state that AST and ALT levels should be determined at baseline as well as periodically (ie, every 2 to 4 weeks) for the first 6 months of therapy and periodically thereafter as deemed clinically relevant by the physician.

Dosage and Administration

The recommended starting dose of tolcapone is 100 mg tid always taken with each dose of levodopa. Increasing the dose to 200 mg tid should only be attempted if there is potential clinical benefit. If there is no clinical response after 3 weeks at 200 mg tid, then tolcapone should be discontinued.

■ Entacapone (Comtan/Comtess)

A peripherally acting COMT inhibitor, entacapone has been shown to increase the elimination half-life of levodopa and to increase "on" and decrease "off" times in patients with levodopa-related fluctuations. A number of studies have demonstrated that the drug:

- Prolongs the effect of levodopa
- Does not increase the magnitude of response to levodopa
- Does not delay patients' response to controlled-release (CR) carbidopa/levodopa.

Entacapone prolongs the availability of levodopa in the plasma and thus to the brain by decreasing peripheral O-methylation and slowing its elimination rate, without affecting the maximum plasma levodopa concentration or time to maximum concentration (**Figure 8.11**).

Two large multicenter studies, conducted under the auspices of the Parkinson Study Group (North America) and the Nordic Study Group (Nordic countries), involved 205 and 171 patients, respectively, with motor fluctuations associated with levodopa therapy (particularly the wearing-off phenomenon) who received either entacapone 200 mg or placebo with each dose of levodopa for 24 weeks.[64,65] The primary measure of efficacy was a change in "on" time while awake, as recorded in patients' daily diaries at 30-minute intervals. Other outcome measures included change in UPDRS scores, "off" time, clinical global scales by patients and investigators, reduction in levodopa dose, and clinical adverse effects. At baseline, patients averaged about 9 to 10 hours (60.5%) of "on" time.

Results of the North American study included[64]:

- Entacapone treatment increased the percent "on" time by 5.0 percentage points compared

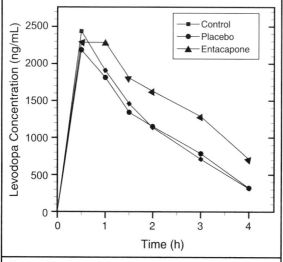

FIGURE 8.11 — Plasma Levodopa Concentrations During Adjunctive Entacapone

Shown here are the mean plasma concentrations of levodopa after an individual oral dose of levodopa (with a levodopa decarboxylase inhibitor) alone (control day) and after 4 weeks of concomitant placebo or entacapone.

Ruottinen HM, Rinne UK. *J Neurol Neurosurg Psychiatry.* 1996;60:36-40.

with placebo, nearly 1 extra hour a day, at weeks 8, 16, and 24.

- The effect of entacapone was more prominent in patients with a smaller baseline "on" time (<55%).
- The effect of entacapone increased as the day wore on.
- At week 24, mean UPDRS scores were improved by approximately 10% among entacapone-treated patients compared with those on placebo.
- On withdrawal of entacapone, patients noted a complete and rapid loss of benefit.

The results of the Nordic study included[65]:

- Entacapone treatment increased "on" time by 1.2 hours (P <0.001)
- Entacapone treatment significantly decreased "off" time by 1.3 hours in an 18-hour day (**Figure 8.12**).
- Withdrawal of entacapone resulted in a significant increase in the duration of "off" time (P <0.001) compared with placebo withdrawal, returning approximately to baseline levels.
- The change in total daily levodopa dose between the two study groups was significant (P <0.001).
- Entacapone-treated patients had a significant reduction in levodopa during treatment.

The efficacy of entacapone on control of motor fluctuations was evaluated in a 6-month, randomized, placebo-controlled trial in 301 levodopa-treated patients, of whom 260 had motor fluctuations.[66] The primary outcome was absolute change in on hours at 6 months compared with baseline. Entacapone significantly (P <0.05) prolonged daily on time by a mean of 1.7 hours from 10.0 at baseline to 11.7 compared with an increase from 9.7 to 10.7 with placebo. The difference versus placebo was greatest in the subgroup of 174 patients taking more than five daily doses of levodopa. UPDRS motor scores improved by 3.3 points with entacapone versus 0.1 points with placebo (P <0.01).

In a subsequent trial, Brooks and colleagues randomized 172 fluctuating and 128 nonfluctuating, levodopa-treated patients to receive entacapone or placebo for 6 months.[67] The primary end point in the nonfluctuating group was the change of the UPDRS ADL score at 4 and 6 months (combined) versus baseline. The primary outcome in the fluctuating group was

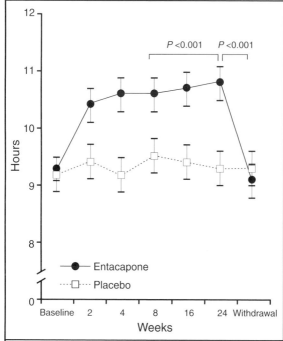

FIGURE 8.12 — Mean "On" Time Measured From Home Diaries in Entacapone Study Group

Mean (± SEM) "on" time from home diaries. Treatment differences were calculated for the last three visits on medication ($P <0.001$). The withdrawal effect difference was calculated for the poststudy visit and the last visit on medication ($P <0.001$).

Adapted from: Rinne UK, et al. *Neurology*. 1998;51:1311.

the proportion of daily on time while awake at 4 and 6 months (combined) versus baseline:

- In the nonfluctuating group, there was a significantly ($P <0.001$) greater improvement in UPDRS ADL scores with entacapone. In addition, the mean daily dose of levodopa increased by 7 mg with entacapone group compared with an increase of 47 mg with placebo ($P < 0.01$).

- In the fluctuating group, entacapone induced a significant increase in mean proportion of daily on time while awake. Mean absolute on time increased by 1.3 hours on entacapone compared with 0.1 hours with placebo ($P < 0.001$).

A recent evidence-based practice parameter published by the American Academy of Neurology states that adjunctive entacapone should be offered to reduce off time (evidence level A).[22]

Although transient dyskinesias and mild nausea are more common with entacapone treatment, this drug is generally well tolerated, with no abnormalities in vital signs or laboratory surveillance tests. The long-term safety and tolerability of entacapone was demonstrated in a 12-month safety study in 326 levodopa-treated patients with and without motor fluctuations, two thirds of whom were randomized to entacapone and one third to placebo.[68] There was no significant difference between entacapone and placebo in the rate of discontinuation due to adverse events (14% vs 11%, respectively). As expected due to dopaminergic enhancement, dyskinesia was a more frequent adverse event with entacapone than with placebo. Entacapone had no adverse effect on hepatic enzymes, ECG, or hemodynamic parameters, and there was no evidence of any toxicity.

Entacapone is also effective in increasing the duration of response to levodopa. **Table 8.6** compares the COMT inhibitor agents.

For patient convenience, a new triple combination tablet (Stalevo) has been developed which contains either:

- 12.5 mg carbidopa/50 mg levodopa/200 mg entacapone (Stalevo 50)
- 25 mg carbidopa/100 mg levodopa/200 mg/ entacapone (Stalevo 100)

TABLE 8.6 — COMT Inhibitors		
	Entacapone	**Tolcapone**
COMT inhibition	Peripheral	Peripheral and central
Dosing	200 mg with every levodopa dose up to 1600 mg entacapone daily	Fixed 100 mg to 200 mg tid
Elimination ($t_{\frac{1}{2}}$)	2 hours	2 hours
Adverse effects	• Nausea • Vomiting • Dyskinesias • Hypotension • Sedation • Headache • Constipation • Diarrhea	• Nausea • Vomiting • Dyskinesias • Sedation • Headache • Severe diarrhea occurring 6 to 8 weeks post-initiation • Increased LFTs*
Abbreviations: COMT, catechol-*O*-methyltransferase; LFT, liver function test; $t_{\frac{1}{2}}$, half-life.		
* Liver-function monitoring required.		

- 37.5 mg carbidopa/150 mg levodopa/200 mg entacapone (Stalevo 150).

The indications for these formulations are the same as those for entacapone, ie, for patients experiencing wearing off with carbidopa/levodopa.

Dosage and Administration

Entacapone should be given 200 mg with each dose of levodopa up to a total daily entacapone dose of 1600 mg.

Carbidopa/Levodopa

The immediate metabolic precursor of dopamine, levodopa (L-3,4-dihydroxyphenylalanine) is transported across the gut wall by a saturable, facilitated carrier system (the aromatic and branched-chain "L" amino acid system).[6] More than 95% of levodopa is rapidly decarboxylated (an overall half-life of 1 hour) to dopamine in the periphery, however, so relatively little unchanged drug reaches the cerebral circulation, and probably <1% actually crosses the blood-brain barrier to permeate striatal tissue. Therefore, levodopa is almost always administered in combination with carbidopa, a peripheral inhibitor of dopa decarboxylase, to increase the fraction of unmetabolized drug available to cross the blood-brain barrier. This combination drug is called Sinemet.

Parcopa (carbidopa/levodopa orally disintegrating tablets) is a unique formulation of carbidopa/levodopa that dissolves rapidly on the tongue. Unlike conventional carbidopa/levodopa tablets, Parcopa uses patented RapiTab technology, an advancement in orally dissolving tablet technology, to deliver an oral dose of medication in a formulation that does not require water. Parcopa is available in the same strengths and has the same dosage schedule as conventional Sinemet (carbidopa/levodopa) tablets. The most common side effects include involuntary movements and nausea.

Equally important, the addition of carbidopa has permitted an approximately 80% reduction in levodopa dosage, thus avoiding most of the nausea, vomiting, hypotension, sinus tachycardia, and orange urine that previously followed conversion of large doses to dopamine by the vascular endothelium. The nausea and vomiting are mediated at the chemoreceptor trigger zone in the area postrema of the medulla, a region with no blood-brain barrier.

Despite levodopa's position as the gold standard for the symptomatic treatment of PD, the timing of its initiation remains somewhat controversial.

■ Levodopa Toxicity

Despite the known benefit of levodopa in reducing the symptoms of Parkinson's disease, there has been concern that it may be toxic to dopaminergic neurons thereby hastening neurodegeneration and progression.[69] Several recent clinical trials in PD patients assessed the possibility that levodopa might be toxic. Two trials that compared levodopa and a dopamine agonist found an increased rate of decline of imaging biomarkers of nigrostriatal function in patients treated with levodopa compared with the dopamine agonist.[70,71] However, since there were no placebo control groups, it is not possible to determine if the difference in the rate of deterioration between these agents was related to a toxic effect of levodopa or a protective effect of the dopamine agonists. Furthermore, these results possibly could be related to pharmacologic differences in the capability of the drugs to induce regulatory changes in components of the nigrostriatal system.[72]

The recently completed Earlier vs Later L-Dopa (ELLDOPA) study compared the rate of disease progression in untreated PD patients randomly assigned to receive one of three doses of levodopa or placebo.[73] The primary end point was the change in UPDRS motor score between untreated baseline and a final visit after 9 months of treatment with study drug and 2 weeks of washout. Neuroimaging studies to determine striatal dopamine-transporter density were also performed in 142 patients at baseline and week 40. The results showed less deterioration from baseline in UPDRS motor score in all three levodopa treatment groups compared with those who received placebo. In contrast, the neuroimaging studies found that levodopa

155

treatment was associated with a greater rate of decline than placebo in a biomarker of nigrostriatal function. Thus, the ELLDOPA study does not resolve the issue of whether or not levodopa is toxic in PD patients.

Compelling evidence for levodopa toxicity has yet to be presented. The treating physician's goal should be to keep patients within the mainstream of life if at all possible. Despite the ongoing debate about when to begin levodopa, once the decision is made, there is little controversy regarding how the drug is to be introduced, titrated, and supplemented with adjunctive agents throughout the course of the disease.

Dosage and Administration

Carbidopa/levodopa treatment is usually started with:

- One half of a 25/100 mg tablet bid after a meal
- Increased by 1/2 tablet per day every 4 to 7 days
- As dosage increases, 25/250 mg tablets can be substituted (only in rare cases are these large doses required). Initiating treatment with the higher dosage may cause:
  - Nausea
  - Dizziness
  - Insomnia
  - Nervousness
  - Vague mental symptoms.

Peripheral dopa decarboxylase is blocked by carbidopa at approximately 70 mg to 100 mg/day. Patients receiving less than that are likely to experience nausea and vomiting.

Realistically, treatment can usually abolish the disability caused by symptoms but cannot be expected to completely relieve symptoms. Therefore, patients must not be allowed to increase dosage on their own. Particularly in the later stages, in which long-term use of levodopa results in dyskinesia, they are likely to mistake the side effect for a worsening of disease and increase the dosage.

Side Effects

The most common serious adverse reactions occurring with carbidopa/levodopa are:

- Choreiform, dystonic, and other involuntary movements
- Mental changes, including paranoid ideation and psychotic episodes
- Nausea
- Cardiac irregularities
- Orthostatic hypotension
- Anorexia
- Vomiting
- Dizziness.

■ Controlled-Release Carbidopa/Levodopa

The mechanism(s) of motor response fluctuations, caused by both peripheral and central pharmacodynamic changes, are not completely understood, but variation in levodopa delivery appears to be a critical factor in their development. Continuous administration of levodopa has been shown to cause fewer behavioral changes and receptor alterations in both animal and clinical studies.

A 35-center, triple-blind, randomized, parallel comparison trial of immediate release (IR) and controlled release (CR) carbidopa/levodopa in untreated PD patients found no significant differences in motor fluctuations over 5 years.[74]

Drugs Under Development

■ Rotigotine

This non-ergoline dopamine agonist is formulated as a transdermal patch for treatment of patients with motor fluctuations. A phase 2 clinical trial demonstrated a significant reduction of levodopa therapy.[75] In a subsequent monotherapy trial, 242 patients with early PD were randomized to receive rotigotine 4.5, 9.0, 13.5, or 18.0 mg or placebo for 11 weeks.[76] Compared with placebo, there were significant (P <0.001), dose-related improvements in the motor and activities of daily living UPDRS scores in the rotigotine 13.5-mg and 18.0-mg groups. Another study in levodopa-treated inpatients with advanced PD found that the rotigotine patch significantly decreased the median levodopa dose without change in UPDRS scores and also resulted in a significant decrease in "off" time.[77]

■ **Istradefylline (KW 6002)**

The adenosine A_{2A} receptor is localized on output neurons in the striatum. The A_{2A} receptor, istradefylline, was studied in a recent small, randomized, placebo-controlled trial of in PD patients with both motor fluctuations and peak-dose dyskinesias. Compared with placebo, treatment with istradefylline resulted in a significant reduction in the proportion of awake time spent in the "off" state as assessed by home diaries compared with an increase with placebo.[78] Dyskinesia severity was unchanged, and there was no difference in change in UPDRS scores. The discontinuation rates in istradefylline- and placebo-treated patient (24% and 20%, respectively) were similar. Nausea was the most common adverse effect with istradefylline. This drug is currently undergoing further clinical evaluations.

■ **Coenzyme Q10**

Coenzyme Q10, or ubiquinone, is a vitamin or vitamin-like substance that functions as the coenzyme for at least three mitochondrial enzymes involved in oxidative phosphorylation and the production of high-energy phosphate and adenosine triphosphate (ATP). Coenzyme Q10 also is a potent antioxidant. Given

158

these properties, it has been suggested that coenzyme Q10 could slow the progression of PD. A double-blind, parallel-group, dose-ranging trial randomized 80 patients with early PD who did not require treatment for their disabilities to receive placebo or coenzyme Q10 at dosages of 300, 600, or 1200 mg/day.[79] Patients were followed for up to 16 months or until disability requiring treatment occurred. The main outcome measure was change from baseline in UPDRS scores. There was a positive linear trend suggesting that all dosages of coenzyme Q10 slowed the development of disabilities as assessed by changes in UPDRS scores. The difference between the coenzyme Q10 1200 mg/day and placebo groups was significant ($P = 0.04$)

REFERENCES

1. Fahn S. Medical treatment of Parkinson's disease. In: 14th Annual Course. A Comprehensive Review of Movement Disorders for the Clinical Practitioner. Vol 1. Aspen, Colo; July 30-August 2, 2004:439-536.

2. Poewe W, Granata R, Geser F. Pharmacologic treatment of Parkinson's disease. In: Watts RL, Koller WC, eds. *Movement Disorders: Neurologic Principles and Practice.* 2nd ed. New York, NY: The McGraw-Hill Companies; 2004:339-358.

3. Chuang C, Waters CH. Initial therapy of Parkinson's disease. In: Samuels M, Feske S, eds. *Office Practice of Neurology.* 2nd ed. Philadelphia, Pa: Churchill Livingstone; 2003:743-748.

4. Waters CH. Advances in managing Parkinson's disease. *Hosp Pract.* 2001;36:27-32, 41.

5. Schrag A, Ben-Shlomo Y, Brown R, Marsden CD, Quinn N. Parkinson's disease revisited – clinical features, natural history, and mortality. *Mov Disord.* 1998;13:885-894.

6. Standaert DG, Young AB. Treatment of central nervous system degenerative disorders: Parkinson's disease. In: Hardman JG, Limbird LE, Molinoff PB, et al, eds. *Goodman and Gilman's The Pharmacological Basis of Therapeutics.* 9th ed. New York, NY: McGraw-Hill; 1996:506-513.

7. Blanpied TA, Boeckman FA, Aizenman E, Johnson JW. Trapping channel block of NMDA-activated responses by amantadine and memantine. *J Neurophysiol.* 1997;77:309-323.

8. Crosby NJ, Deane KH, Clarke CE. Amantadine in Parkinson's disease. *Cochrane Database Syst Rev.* 2003;(1): CD003468.

9. Crosby NJ, Deane KH, Clarke CE. Amantadine for dyskinesia in Parkinson's disease. *Cochrane Database Syst Rev.* 2003;(2):CD003467.

10. Thomas A, Iacono D, Luciano AL, Armellino K, Di Iorio A, Onofrj M. Duration of amantadine benefit in dyskinesia of severe Parkinson's disease. *J Neurol Neurosurg Psychiatry.* 2004;75:141-143.

11. The Parkinson Study Group. Effect of deprenyl on the progression of disability in early Parkinson's disease. *N Engl J Med.* 1989;321:1364-1371.

12. Parkinson Study Group. Impact of deprenyl and tocopherol treatment on Parkinson's disease in DATATOP subjects not requiring levodopa. *Ann Neurol.* 1996;39:29-36.

13. Parkinson Study Group. Impact of deprenyl and tocopherol treatment on Parkinson's disease in DATATOP patients requiring levodopa. *Ann Neurol.* 1996;39:37-45.

14. Giladi N, McDermott MP, Fahn S, et al. Freezing of gait in PD: prospective assessment in the DATATOP cohort. *Neurology.* 2001;56:1712-1721.

15. Koller WC. Neuroprotective therapy for Parkinson's disease. *Exp Neurol.* 1997;144:24-28.

16. Langston JW, Tanner CM. Selegiline and Parkinson's disease: it's deja vu-again. *Neurology.* 2000;55:1770-1771.

17. Goetz CG, Poewe W, Rascol O, Sampaio C. Evidence-based medical review update: pharmacological and surgical treatments of Parkinson's disease: 2001 to 2004. *Mov Disord.* 2005;20:523-539.

18. Lees AJ. Comparison of therapeutic effects and mortality data of levodopa and levodopa combined with selegiline in patients with early, mild Parkinson's disease. Parkinson's Disease Research Group of the United Kingdom. *BMJ.* 1995; 311:1602-1607.

19. Olanow CW, Myllyla VV, Sotaniemi KA, et al. Effect of selegiline on mortality in patients with Parkinson's disease: a meta-analysis. *Neurology.* 1998;51:825-830.

20. Donnan PT, Steinke DT, Stubbings C, Davey PG, MacDonald TM. Selegiline and mortality in subjects with Parkinson's disease: a longitudinal community study. *Neurology.* 2000;55:1785-1789.

21. Ives NJ, Stow RL, Marro J, et al. Monomine oxidase type B inhibitors in early Parkinson's disease: meta-analysis for 17 randomized trials involving 3525 patients. *BMJ.* 2004;329: 593.

22. Pahwa R, Factor SA, Lyons KE, et al; Quality Standards Subcommittee of the American Academy of Neurology. Practice Parameter: treatment of Parkinson disease with motor fluctuations and dyskinesia (an evidence-based review): report of the Quality Standards Subcommittee of the American Academy of Neurology. *Neurology.* 2006;66:983-995.

23. Clarke A, Johnson ES, Mallard N, et al. A new low-dose formulation of selegiline: clinical efficacy, patient preference and selectivity for MAO-B inhibition. *J Neural Transm.* 2003;110:1257-1271.

24. Waters CH, Sethi KD, Hauser RA, Molho E, Bertoni JM; Zydis Selegiline Study Group. Zydis selegiline reduces off time in Parkinson's disease patients with motor fluctuations: a 3-month, randomized, placebo-controlled study. *Mov Disord.* 2004;19:426-432,

25. Ondo WG. Pooled analysis of two identical phase 3 studies of novel selegiline preparation as adjunctive therapy for Parkinson's disease. *Mov Disord.* 2006;21:S126.

8

26. Maruyama W, Yamamoto T, Kitani K, Carrillo MC, Youdim M, Naoi M. Mechanism underlying anti-apoptotic activity of a (-)deprenyl-related propargylamine, rasagiline. *Mech Ageing Dev.* 2000;116:181-191.

27. Abu-Raya S, Blaugrund E, Trembovler V, Shilderman-Bloch E, Shohami E, Lazarovici P. Rasagiline, a monoamine oxidase-B inhibitor, protects NGF-differentiated PC12 cells against oxygen-glucose deprivation. *J Neurosci Res.* 1999; 58:456-463.

28. Abu-Raya S, Tabakman R, Blaugrund E, Trembovler V, Lazarovici P. Neuroprotective and neurotoxic effects of monoamine oxidase-B inhibitors and derived metabolites under ischemia in PC12 cells. *Eur J Pharmacol.* 2002;434: 109-116.

29. Stern MB, Marek KL, Friedman J, et al. Double-blind, randomized, controlled trial of rasagiline as monotherapy in early Parkinson's disease patients. *Mov Disord.* 2004;19:916-923.

30. Parkinson Study Group. A controlled trial of rasagiline in early Parkinson disease: the TEMPO Study. *Arch Neurol.* 2002;59:1937-1943.

31. Parkinson Study Group. A controlled, randomized, delayed-start study of rasagiline in early Parkinson disease. *Arch Neurol.* 2004;61:561-566.

32. Parkinson Study Group. A randomized placebo-controlled trial of rasagiline in levodopa-treated patients with Parkinson disease and motor fluctuations: the PRESTO study. *Arch Neurol.* 2005;62:241-248.

33. Rascol O, Brooks DJ, Melamed E, et al; LARGO study group. Rasagiline as an adjunct to levodopa in patients with Parkinson's disease and motor fluctuations (LARGO, Lasting effect in Adjunct therapy with Rasagiline Given Once daily, study): a randomised, double-blind, parallel-group trial. *Lancet.* 2005;365:947-954.

34. Oertel WH, Wolters E, Sampaio C, et al. Pergolide versus levodopa monotherapy in early Parkinson's disease patients: The PELMOPET study. *Mov Disord.* 2006;21:343-353.

35. Baseman DG, O'Suilleabhain PE, Reimold SC, Laskar SR, Baseman JG, Dewey RG Jr. Pergolide use in Parkinson's disease is associated with cardiac valve regurgitation. *Neurology.* 2004;63:301-304.

36. Rinne UK, Bracco F, Chouza C, et al. Early treatment of Parkinson's disease with cabergoline delays the onset of motor complications. Results of a double-blind levodopa controlled trial. *Drugs.* 1998;55(suppl 1):23-30.

37. Horvath J, Fross RD, Kleiner-Fisman G, et al. Severe multivalvular heart disease: a new complication of the ergot derivative dopamine agonists. *Mov Disord.* 2004;19:656-662.

38. Mierau J, Schneider FJ, Ensinger HA, Chio CL, Lajiness ME, Huff RM. Pramipexole binding and activation of cloned and expressed dopamine D_2, D_3 and D_4 receptors. *Eur J Pharmacol.* 1995;290:29-36.

39. Shannon KM, Bennett JP Jr, Friedman JH. Efficacy of pramipexole, a novel dopamine agonist, as monotherapy in mild to moderate Parkinson's disease. The Pramipexole Study Group. *Neurology.* 1997;49:724-728.

40. Parkinson Study Group. Safety and efficacy of pramipexole in early Parkinson disease. A randomized dose-ranging study. *JAMA.* 1997;278:125-130.

41. Parkinson Study Group. Pramipexole vs levodopa as initial treatment for Parkinson's disease. A randomized controlled trial. *JAMA.* 2000;284:1931-1938.

42. Holloway RG, Shoulson I, Fahn S, et al; Parkinson Study Group. Pramipexole vs levodopa as initial treatment for Parkinson's disease. *Arch Neurol.* 2004;61:1044-1053.

43. Lieberman A, Ranhosky A, Korts D. Clinical evaluation of pramipexole in advanced Parkinson's disease: results of a double-blind, placebo-controlled, parallel-group study. *Neurology.* 1997;49:162-168.

44. Weiner WJ, Factor SA, Jankovic J, et al. The long-term safety and efficacy of pramipexole in advanced Parkinson's disease. *Parkinsonism Relat Dis.* 2001;7:115-120.

45. Moller JC, Oertel WH, Koster J, Pezzoli G, Provinciali L. Long-term efficacy and safety of pramipexole in advanced Parkinson's disease: results from a European multicenter trial. *Mov Disord.* 2005;20:602-610.

46. Wong KS, Lu CS, Shan DE, Yang CC, Tsoi TH, Mok V. Efficacy, safety, and tolerability of pramipexole in untreated and levodopa-treated patients with Parkinson's disease. *J Neurol Sci.* 2003;216:81-87.

47. Pogarell O, Gasser T, van Hilten JJ, et al. Pramipexole in patients with Parkinson's disease and marked drug resistant tremor: a randomised, double blind, placebo controlled multicentre study. *J Neurol Neurosurg Psychiatry.* 2002;72: 713-720.

48. Frucht S, Rogers JD, Greene PE, Gordon MF, Fahn S. Falling asleep at the wheel: motor vehicle mishaps in persons taking pramipexole and ropinirole. *Neurology.* 1999;52: 1908-1910.

49. Tulloch IF. Pharmacologic profile of ropinirole: a nonergoline dopamine agonist. *Neurology.* 1997;49(1 suppl 1):S58-S62.

50. Rascol O. Ropinirole: clinical profile. In: Olanow CW, Obeso JA, eds. *Beyond the Decade of the Brain.* Vol 2. Royal Tunbridge Wells, UK: Wells Medical Limited; 1997:163-175.

51. Adler CH, Sethi KD, Hauser RA, et al. Ropinirole for the treatment of early Parkinson's disease. The Ropinirole Study Group. *Neurology.* 1997;49:393-399.

52. Rascol O, Brooks DJ, Korczyn AD, De Deyn PP, Clarke CE, Lang AE. A five-year study of the incidence of dyskinesia in patients with early Parkinson's disease who were treated with ropinirole or levodopa. 056 Study group. *N Engl J Med.* 2000;342:1484-1491.

53. Korczyn AD, Brunt ER, Larsen JP, Nagy Z, Poewe WH, Ruggieri S. A 3-year randomized trial of ropinirole and bromocriptine in early Parkinson's disease. *Neurology.* 1999;53:364-370.

54. Sethi KD, O'Brien CF, Hammerstad JP, et al. Ropinirole for the treatment of early Parkinson disease: a 12-month experience. Ropinirole Study group. *Arch Neurol*. 1998;55:1211-1216.

55. Korczyn AD, Keens J, Macrae S. The safety and efficacy of ropinirole as early therapy in elderly patients with Parkinson's disease. *Neurology*. 2000;54(suppl 3):A90. Abstract.

56. Rascol O, Lees AJ, Senard JM, Pirtosek Z, Montastruc JL, Fuell D. Ropinirole in the treatment of levodopa-induced motor fluctuations in patients with Parkinson's disease. *Clin Neuropharmacol*. 1996;19:234-245.

57. Lieberman A, Olanow CW, Sethi K, et al. A multicenter trial of ropinirole as adjunct treatment for Parkinson's disease. *Neurology*. 1998;51:1057-1062.

58. Goetz CG, Blasucci L, Stebbins GT. Switching dopamine agonists in advanced Parkinson's disease. Is rapid titration preferable to slow? *Neurology*. 1999;52:1227-1229.

59. Kurth MC, Adler CH, Hilaire MS, et al. Tolcapone improves motor function and reduces levodopa requirement in patients with Parkinson's disease experiencing motor fluctuations: a multicenter, double-blind, randomized, placebo-controlled trial. Tolcapone Fluctuator Study Group I. *Neurology*. 1997;48:81-87.

60. Waters CH, Kurth M, Bailey P, et al. Tolcapone in stable Parkinson's disease: efficacy and safety of long-term treatment. The Tolcapone Stable Study group. *Neurology*. 1997; 49:665-671.

61. Parkinson Study Group. Entacapone improves motor fluctuations in patients in levodopa-treated Parkinson's disease patients. *Ann Neurol*. 1997;42:747-755.

62. Rajput AH, Martin W, Saint-Hilaire MH, Dorflinger E, Pedder S. Tolcapone improves motor function in parkinsonian patients with the "wearing-off" phenomenon: a double-blind, placebo-controlled, multicenter trial. *Neurology*. 1997;49:1066-1071.

8

63. Keating GM, Lyseng-Williamson KA. Tolcapone: a review of its use in the management of Parkinson's disease. *CNS Drugs*. 2005;19:165-184.

64. Baas H, Beiske AG, Ghika J, et al. Catechol-O-methyl-transferase inhibition with tolcapone reduces the "wearing off" phenomenon and levodopa requirements in fluctuating parkinsonian patients. *J Neurol Neurosurg Psychiatry*. 1997; 63:421-428.

65. Rinne UK, Larsen JP, Siden A, Worm-Petersen J. Entacapone enhances the response to levodopa in parkinsonian patients with motor fluctuations. Nomecomt Study group. *Neurology*. 1998;51:1309-1314.

66. Poewe WH, Deuschl G, Gordin A, Kultalahti ER, Leinonen M; Celomen Study Group. Efficacy and safety of entacapone in Parkinson's disease patients with suboptimal levodopa response: a 6-month randomized placebo-controlled double-blind study in Germany and Austria (Celomen study). *Acta Neurol Scand*. 2002;105:245-255.

67. Brooks DJ, Sagar H; UK-Irish Entacapone Study Group. Entacapone is beneficial in both fluctuating and non-fluctuating patients with Parkinson's disease: a randomised, placebo controlled, double blind, six month study. *J Neurol Neurosurg Psychiatry*. 2003;74:1071-1079.

68. Myllyla VV, Kultalahti ER, Haapaniemi H, Leinonen M; FILOMEN Study Group. Twelve-month safety of entacapone in patients with Parkinson's disease. *Eur J Neurol*. 2001;8: 53-60.

69. Olanow CW, Agid Y, Mizumo Y, et al. Levodopa in the treatment of Parkinson's disease: current controversies. *Mov Disord*. 2004;19:997-1005.

70. Parkinson Study Group. Dopamine transporter brain imaging to assess the effects of pramipexole vs levodopa on Parkinson disease progression. *JAMA*. 2002;287:1653-1661.

71. Whone A, Watts R, Stoessl J, et al; REAL-PET Study group. Slower progression of Parkinson's disease with ropinirole versus levodopa: the REAL-PET Study. *Ann Neurol*. 2003; 54:93-101.

72. Ahlskog JE. Slowing Parkinson's disease progression: recent dopamine agonist trials. *Neurology.* 2003;60:381-389.

73. Fahn S, Oakes D, Shoulson I, et al; Parkinson Study Group. Levodopa and the progression of Parkinson's disease. *N Engl J Med.* 2004;351:2498-2508.

74. Koller WC, Hutton JT, Tolosa E, Capilldeo R. Immediate-release and controlled-release carbidopa/levodopa in PD: a 5-year randomized multicenter study. Carbidopa/Levodopa Study Group. *Neurology.* 1999;53:1012-1019.

75. Hutton JT, Metman LV, Chase TN, et al. Transdermal dopaminergic D_2 receptor agonist therapy in Parkinson's disease with N-0923 TDS: a double-blind, placebo-controlled study. *Mov Disord.* 2001;16:459-463.

76. The Parkinson Study Group. A controlled trial of rotigotine monotherapy in early Parkinson's disease. *Arch Neurol.* 2003;60:1721-1728.

77. Metman LV, Gillespie M, Farmer C, et al. Continuous transdermal dopaminergic stimulation in advanced Parkinson's disease. *Clin Neuropharmacol.* 2001;24:163-169.

78. Hauser RA, Hubble JP, Truong DD; Istradefylline US-001 Study Group. Randomized trial of the adenosine A(2A) receptor antagonist istradefylline in advanced PD. *Neurology.* 2003;61:297-303.

79. Shults CW, Oakes D, Kieburtz K, et al; Parkinson Study group. Effects of coenzyme Q10 in early Parkinson disease: evidence of slowing of the functional decline. *Arch Neurol.* 2002;59:1541-1550.

9 Complications of Parkinson's Disease and Its Therapy

Levodopa remains the most effective drug for symptomatic treatment of Parkinson's disease (PD), but as the disease progresses, the emergence of motor fluctuations and dyskinesias limits its continuing usefulness. Therefore, the essentially inevitable emergence of treatment-related motor complications of later-stage PD becomes very much a part of everyday management and shapes therapeutic interventions. A host of other problems (behavioral, autonomic, and sleep) can significantly alter that treatment plan. Both motor and nonmotor complications will be summarized here.

Levodopa-Related Motor Complications

The natural progression of PD typically begins with an insidious onset of symptoms, such as decreased arm swing, rest tremor, shuffling gait, or bradykinesia, followed by improvement with initiation of dopaminergic therapy. This "honeymoon" period, however, gradually comes to an end with the emergence of shortening of response to levodopa, wearing-off effect, peak-dose dyskinesia, and ultimately, unpredictable response without obvious relationship to levodopa dosing, the so-called "on-off" effect (**Figure 9**.1).[1]

■ Factors Influencing Levodopa Efficacy

Motor fluctuations are determined by peripheral and central levodopa pharmacokinetics and central pharmacodynamic influences (**Table 9**.1).[2] Gastrointes-

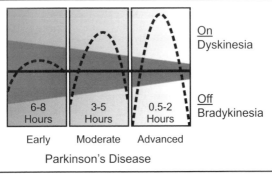
tinal (GI) activity is crucial to the delivery of levodopa to the brain. Since absorption of levodopa occurs mostly in the duodenum and jejunum, erratic gastric

emptying is a controlling factor. Under certain conditions, it may result in lower plasma levodopa concentrations or may be responsible for some biphasic absorption patterns. Factors, such as increased gastric acidity, antiparkinsonian drugs (primarily anticholinergics), and food, affect gastric emptying.

Levodopa is transported from gut to blood and across the blood-brain barrier on the large, neutral amino acid carrier system. With normal food intake, concentrations of neutral amino acids in blood are near saturation for blood-brain transport. Therefore, food-derived amino acids have the potential to interfere with levodopa transport. For example, protein loads with significant amounts of neutral amino acids can interfere with levodopa uptake. In addition, physical activity may reduce mesenteric blood flow, decreasing levodopa absorption and worsening fluctuations.

Factors affecting central pharmacokinetics include pulsatile delivery of levodopa to striatal receptors and impaired storage capacity of dopamine, caused by the progressive loss of nigral neurons. During the first few years of levodopa therapy, symptoms tend to improve and remain under stable control with infrequent dosing, two or three times a day. The remaining nigrostriatal neurons provide adequate dopamine storage capacity, and the brain retains its ability to buffer swings in cerebral levodopa availability. Within 3 to 5 years, however, with increased nigral cell death, there is a gradual but unpredictable tendency for the early, smooth response to levodopa to give way to the nonphysiologic, short-duration response, which emerges as a subtle-later, a more pronounced-pattern of "wearing off" and "on/off" motor fluctuations complicated by abnormal involuntary movements or dyskinesias (**Figure 9.1**).

There are several hypotheses for the development of motor fluctuations. In a recent review, Olanow and colleagues consider the controversy over the potential of levodopa to exert toxic effects on dopaminergic neurons via generation of reactive oxygen species.[3] Although levodopa has been shown to be toxic to cultured dopamine neurons, the authors note that clinical trials have not clarified this question. They do point out that the concentrations of levodopa used in most tissue culture studies was up to 5-fold higher than the plasma concentrations achieved in treated PD patients.

An alternate hypothesis for the development of motor fluctuations was proposed by Metman, who suggested that nonphysiological, intermittent dopaminergic stimulation (mostly by levodopa since fewer fluctuations are seen with dopamine agonists) activates signal transduction pathways in the striatum.[4] This may lead to enhanced N-methyl-D-aspartate (NMDA) receptor subunit phosphorylation, and the receptors become more sensitive to glutamatergic corticostriatal input. This translates clinically to motor fluctuations and dyskinesias. This also explains the benefit of the NMDA receptor antagonist amantadine in controlling these difficulties. Ultimately, however, the most important factor in preventing motor fluctuations is prevention of ongoing degeneration.

Risk Factors

The frequency (hence risk) of levodopa-related motor complications is dependent on a number of risk factors, such as the age at onset of the disease and initiation of levodopa therapy, duration of treatment, total daily dose, and other factors.

The effect of age at onset on motor complications is illustrated by a study by Silver and associates who compared 88 patients with young-onset PD (onset between 20 and 40 years) with 110 late-onset PD patients (onset at 60 years or older).[5] Significantly more levodopa-treated young-onset patients developed rigidity, wearing-off phenomena, and dyskinesias (**Table 9.2**).

TABLE 9.2 — Presenting Features and Levodopa-Related Motor Complications in Young vs Late Onset Parkinson's Disease

Symptom	Presenting (%)		P Value
	Young Onset (20-40 yrs) n = 88	Late Onset (≥60 yrs) n = 110	
Tremor	59.1	65.5	NS
Bradykinesia	10.2	14.5	NS
Rigidity	18.2	8.2	0.051
Postural instability	3.4	13.6	0.013
Gait difficulty	14.8	28.2	0.026
Wearing off	73.8	36.8	0.00001
Wearing-off dystonia	25.8	5.3	0.0003
L-Dopa dyskinesias	69.2	41.1	0.0007

Adapted from: Silver GA, et al. *Mov Disord.* 2004;19(suppl 9):S264.

9

There are many apparent discrepancies in the frequency of motor complications between the different studies, perhaps the most important of which is a difference in definitions of the thresholds for recognizing motor complications.[1] A retrospective review of 74 publications dating from 1966 through 2000 with adequate data related to frequency of levodopa-induced fluctuations and dyskinesias concluded that patients from the pre-levodopa era experienced dyskinesias much earlier during levodopa treatment than patients during the current era, possibly because of longer durations of preexisting PD.[6] The authors also found that after 5 years of levodopa therapy, about 40% of current-era patients experience motor fluctuations and the same number experience dyskinesias.

In a large, prospective study, 352 "de novo" patients originally enrolled in the Deprenyl and Tocopherol Antioxidative Therapy of Parkinsonism (DATATOP) protocol experienced the following complications after 20.5 ± 8.8 months of levodopa therapy: about half developed wearing off, one third developed dyskinesia, and 10% developed severe on-off fluctuations.[7] However, in the CR Five-Year International Response Fluctuation Study (CR FIRST), in which standard and CR Sinemet were compared, only 22% of the patients developed fluctuations or dyskinesias during a 5-year prospective follow-up.[8] However, when patients are carefully observed, a majority of them develop motor fluctuations and dyskinesias even during the first year of levodopa therapy.[9]

The daily dosage of levodopa is also a risk factor for the development of dyskinesias. For example, in the Earlier vs Later L-Dopa (ELLDOPA) trial that evaluated the effects of levodopa on progression of PD in 361 patients with no prior anti-PD treatment and not requiring symptomatic therapy were randomized to placebo or levodopa at 150, 300, or 600 mg/day for 40 weeks, followed by a 2-week washout.[10] Wearing off and dyskinesias were significantly more common in the highest-dose group.

A genetic predisposition for the development of levodopa-related complications could explain the marked inter-subject heterogeneity of response to levodopa. Although several studies found an association between certain polymorphisms of the dopamine receptor genes and high risk of early development of motor complications in levodopa-treated patients, other studies found no such associations.[1]

■ Motor Fluctuations: Characteristics and Management
Clinical Characteristics

The wearing-off phenomenon (**Table 9.3**) is the most common form of clinical fluctuation, and is characterized by end-of-dose deterioration and recurrence of parkinsonian symptoms as a result of shorter (sometimes only 1 to 2 hours) duration of benefit after a given dose of levodopa. The patient experiences a return of parkinsonian symptoms and signs, such as bradykinesia, tremor, rigidity, difficulty arising from a chair, getting in and out of a car, or freezing. Although freezing is a common parkinsonian sign during the "off" state, it may occur even when the patient

TABLE 9.3 — Levodopa-Related Motor Fluctuations
• Wearing off: – Gradual, sudden   – Predictable (related to meals, exercise, rest)   – Unpredictable   • On-off (random "yo-yoing")   • Delayed on   • No on (dose failure)   • Freezing (off, on – may not be related to levodopa)
Adapted from: Jankovic J. *Mov Disord.* 2005;20(suppl):S11-S16.

is "on" ("on freezing").[1] Besides the return of parkinsonian symptoms, some patients experience "off dyskinesias," most frequently "off dystonia." The fluctuations may have a gradual or sudden onset, be predictably associated with activities such as meals, exercise or rest, or be totally unpredictable. On-off fluctuations (random "yo-yo-ing") are characterized by sudden, unpredictable shifts between undertreated and overtreated states. Furthermore, patients may report a 20-minute or so worsening of symptoms after taking levodopa. This seems to be a transient effect that does not require treatment. Finally, the drug-failure response to levodopa is a phenomenon that occurs in the late afternoon and may be related to poor gastric emptying and inadequate absorption.

In addition to motor fluctuations, patients may experience sensory, psychiatric, and autonomic fluctuations (discussed below) during "off" periods and, if not recognized as part of the levodopa response pattern, may result in the ordering of unnecessary diagnostic tests. For example, many patients who complain of shortness of breath undergo extensive pulmonary evaluations only to discover that this symptom is actually caused by the levodopa wearing-off phenomenon.

Management

Growing preclinical and clinical evidence suggests that the development and severity of motor fluctuations is influenced both by PD severity and pulsatile stimulation of striatal dopamine receptors.[4] Thus current management of motor fluctuations rests primarily on strategies to prolong the effects of dopaminergic stimulation. This is accomplished either through the use of long-acting dopaminergic drugs or prolongation of the effects of levodopa.

Dietary alterations can be a useful first step in management of motor fluctuations since a patient's responsiveness to levodopa can be affected by timing of meals in relation to the medication schedule, gastric emptying time, and high-protein meals.[11] When taken in the fed state, levodopa concentrations may be delayed, and competition with dietary amino acids can interfere with transportation of levodopa across the intestinal mucosa and the blood-brain barrier. The former situation can be addressed by timing dosages of levodopa to the symptoms manifested and meal schedule. Symptom diaries kept by the patient or caregiver can be used to characterize the patient's medication response patterns. For patients who demonstrate extreme sensitivity and delayed response after high-protein meals, a nonprotein breakfast and lunch, and higher protein dinner may be prescribed.

Pharmacologic strategies for managing *wearing-off phenomena* focus on adjusting the medication dose for optimal effect. In order to "smooth" and sustain plasma levels, sustained-release carbidopa/levodopa preparations may be substituted in part or totally for the immediate-release levodopa previously used. However, when switching from immediate release to the sustained-release preparations, the levodopa dose must be increased. Reduced bioavailability from a sustained-release preparation requires that the total daily levodopa dose be about 1-1/3 times that from an immediate-release preparation for most patients.

Patients with levodopa-induced motor fluctuations often respond well to adjunctive therapy with other anti-parkinsonian agents. The American Academy of Neurology recently published an evidence-based practice parameter for the treatment of motor fluctuations and dyskinesia.[12] The recommendations are summarized in **Table 9.4**. Detailed discussions of the individual medications, including the recently approved buccal formulation of selegiline (zydis selegiline) and the specific MAO-B inhibitor rasagiline, are provided in Chapter 8, *Treatment*.

TABLE 9.4 — Evidence-Based Recommendations for Treatment of Patients With Parkinson's Disease With Levodopa-Induced Motor Fluctuations

Should Be Offered to Reduce "Off" Time (Evidence Level A) • Rasagiline • Entacapone
Should Be Considered to Reduce "Off" Time (Evidence Level B) • Pergolide • Pramipexole • Ropinirole • Tolcapone
May Be Considered to Reduce "Off" Time (Evidence Level C) • Apomorphine • Cabergoline • Selegiline
Note: Available evidence does not establish superiority of one medicine over another in reducing off time (evidence level B).
Adapted from: Pahwa R, et al. *Neurology*. 2006;66:983-995.

Subcutaneous apomorphine has long been used to reduce the duration of "off" periods in patients with motor fluctuations. Its onset of action is 3 to 20 minutes and its duration of action is 20 to 40 minutes. To determine the therapeutic dose, an apomorphine challenge must be conducted after the patient is evaluated for cardiac dysrhythmias and pretreated with domperidone or trimethobenzamide (tigan) (United States) for 3 days.[11] A pre-filled variable dose pen injector is available to facilitate patient self-administration. Sublingual and transdermal delivery routes for apomorphine are under development.[13,14]

Rotigotine (formerly known as N-9023 TDS), a non-ergoline dopamine agonist on D_3/D_2 receptors, is also being developed as a transdermal patch for treatment of patients with motor fluctuations. A phase 2 clinical trial demonstrated a significant benefit with this therapy.[15] Adverse effects included nausea, hallucinations, and somnolence. However, the incidence of adverse effects was lower with the patch than typically expected with oral dopamine agonists. Another study in levodopa-treated inpatients with advanced PD found that the rotigotine patch significantly decreased the median levodopa dose without change in UPDRS scores and there was also a significant decrease in "off" time.[16]

Because they are sudden and unpredictable, *"on-off" fluctuations* are difficult to treat. Smooth activation of striatal dopamine receptors throughout the day is required to prevent these fluctuations. To avoid the "off" state, some patients self medicate and increase their medication dosage. This results in dyskinesias alternating with "off." Consequently, there is little good "on" time.

The addition of, or an increase in the dosage of, a dopamine agonist or increased doses of levodopa can be tried; however, most pharmacologic interventions that improve the "on" time will increase dyskinesias. Changing to liquefied carbidopa/levodopa in small doses throughout the day can be considered in patients with severe fluctuations that cannot be managed with other measures. Liquefied carbidopa/levodopa may allow more consistent and reliable control. Close titration is possible with this strategy and may result in less "off" time and potentially fewer dyskinesias. This option, though, is viable only in highly motivated patients who are willing to accept the inconvenience of very frequent dosing and daily preparation. Because commercial products are unavailable, the solution must be prepared daily, as follows:

9

- Pulverize 10 tablets of 25/100 mg IR carbidopa/levodopa and 2 g of ascorbic acid.
- Combine the powder with 1 liter tap water.
- Administer in small doses at 60- to 90-minute intervals, titrated to response; total daily dose should equal that prescribed in tablet formulation.

As noted above, *freezing* may occur during either "on" or "off" states. "Off" freezing is managed by keeping the patients from turning "off." "On" freezing is poorly understood and does not respond readily to levodopa. That freezing may reflect a deficiency in the neurotransmitter, norepinephrine, has been suggested, but treatment of the deficiency with a norepinephrine precursor has proved unsatisfactory. One pilot study reported some benefit of botulinum toxin injections into the calf muscles.[17]

Other suggestions to overcome freezing include auditory, visual (parallel lines on the walking surface), and proprioceptive cues. In one study, an inverted walking stick helped some patients.

■ Dyskinesias: Characteristics and Management
Clinical Characteristics

The most frequent forms of dyskinesia (**Table 9.5**) include stereotypies, chorea, ballism, dystonia, and myoclonus.[1] Although these involuntary movements can be quite violent and disabling, many patients prefer being "on" with dyskinesia than being "off" without dyskinesia. Studies of patients during periods of dyskinesias suggest that levodopa-induced dyskinesias usually start in the foot, ipsilateral to the side most affected by PD.[18,19]

Peak-dose dyskinesia, the most common type of dyskinesia, usually manifests as stereotypic, choreic, or ballistic movements involving the head, trunk, and limbs, and occasionally, the respiratory muscles.[1] The so-called *diphasic dyskinesia* that occurs as plasma levodopa levels are rising or falling, occurs in about 15% to 20% of patients chronically treated with levodopa. In contrast to the more frequent peak-dose dyskinesias, characterized by the sequence of **i**mprovement-**d**yskinesia-**i**mprovement (I-D-I), the diphasic response is characterized by **d**yskinesia-**i**mprovement-**d**yskinesia (D-I-D).

Levodopa-related *dystonia* tends to occur when plasma, and presumably brain, levels are either rising or falling.[1] Probably the most common form of dystonia in levodopa-treated PD patients consists of wearing off, including morning or nocturnal, and painful foot cramps.

Management

Treatment of *peak-dose dyskinesia* consists of reducing individual levodopa doses. However, reducing the amount in an individual dose decreases the duration of benefit and can result in more severe "off" states. Therefore, patients may require more frequent doses of the lower dosages of levodopa. Sustained-release carbidopa/levodopa preparations (Sinemet CR) can be used to lower peak plasma levodopa levels, thereby decreasing dyskinesias. However, the dyskinesias may have a longer duration due to the slow fall in plasma levodopa levels. Frequent dosing of sustained-release levodopa preparations may also increase dyskinesias at the end of the day due to sustained levodopa plasma levels. Patients who do well for most of the day on sustained-release carbidopa/levodopa but have trouble with early-morning akinesia may benefit from taking the immediate-release along with the sustained-release dose first thing in the morning. This regimen jump-starts the day for these patients, preparing them physically for normal activities.

Addition of a dopamine agonist or a COMT inhibitor may allow for reduced levodopa dosage without compromising symptomatic control. Adjunctive use of the glutamate antagonist amantadine also may allow smaller and more frequent doses of carbidopa/levodopa.[29,30] Therapy is initiated with 100 mg bid and increased stepwise to 200 mg bid, as needed. However, according to a recent report, the antidyskinetic benefit lasts <8 months.[22] The atypical neuroleptic clozapine has been shown to suppress levodopa-related dyskinesias while increasing "on" time.[23,24] Propranolol has also been reported to reduce dyskinesias.[25] Unfortunately, there is no reported effective treatment for diphasic dyskinesia, although higher doses of levodopa have been recommended.[26] Ultimately some of these patients may need to be referred for surgery to control these movements.

Nonmotor Symptoms and Complications

The importance and impact of the nonmotor manifestations of PD (**Table 9.6**) are being increasingly rec-

TABLE 9.6 — Nonmotor Complications of Parkinson's Disease

Neuropsychiatric
- Cognitive impairment and dementia
- Psychosis
- Depression
- Apathy
- Anxiety

Autonomic Dysfunction
- Orthostatic hypotension
- Gastrointestinal
- Genitourinary
- Sweating

Sleep Disorders
- Insomnia
- Excessive daytime sleepiness
- Rapid eye movement-sleep behavior disorder (RBD)
- Restless legs syndrome
- Sleep apnea

Sensory Disorders
- Akathisia
- Olfaction

ognized. It has been estimated that 60% of PD patients have two or more nonmotor symptoms, and 25% have four or more.[27] This presents a challenge in the overall management of PD patients since nonmotor manifestations respond much less consistently to dopaminergic medications than motor complications and often are sources of dissatisfaction for patients. However, various therapeutic strategies, discussed below, have been developed to deal with the nonmotor signs and symptoms of PD.

■ Neuropsychiatric Symptoms
Dementia

Dementia is one of the most feared complications of PD since it can result in loss of intellectual facilities and increased caregiver burden. In addition, it can limit the amount of medications PD patients may take for their motor symptoms, with a resultant loss of benefit. These patients respond poorly to levodopa and experience frequent side effects, and their disability progresses rapidly. Finally, dementia is associated with poorer prognosis for survival in PD patients.[28]

The dementia associated with PD has been estimated to affect 20% to 40% of patients if one accepts the DSM-IV definition (ie, cognitive dysfunction severe enough to cause functional impairment).[29,30] The prevalence is higher in older patients and rare in those with young-onset disease. Distinctions are often blurred between Parkinson's dementia, Alzheimer's with parkinsonism, and dementia with Lewy bodies (see Chapter 7, *Diagnosis*). Until a disease-specific biologic maker that differentiates the various neurodegenerative disorders is identified, the clinical diagnosis of the various dementing diseases will continue to present a diagnostic challenge.

Management

Before treating dementia in a patient with PD, it is crucial to eliminate all reversible causes, such as subdural hematoma, vitamin B_{12} deficiency, hypothyroidism, normal-pressure hydrocephalus, and mass lesions. If cognitive fluctuations are prominent, evidence of superimposed infection, seizures, transient ischemic attacks, or orthostatic hypotension should be sought.

Once identifiable factors have been eliminated, all medications should be reassessed. Antiparkinsonian agents should be tapered and withdrawn in order of greatest propensity to cause cognitive side effects. Fortunately, this list happens to be in reverse order of antiparkinsonian efficacy:

1. Anticholinergic agents
2. Amantadine

3. Dopamine agonists
4. Levodopa (and its promoters, COMT and MAO-B inhibitors)

Eventually, this stepwise tapering or withdrawal of antiparkinsonian medications will result in an unacceptable deterioration in control of PD symptoms. At this point, one should consider prescribing agents used for symptomatic treatment of cognitive deficits in patients with Alzheimer's disease, such as:

- Donepezil (Aricept)
- Galantamine (Razadyne, formerly Reminyl)
- Rivastigmine (Exelon)
- Tacrine (Cognex).

Although three of these agents are not approved by the FDA for use in PD patients, rivastigmine was recently approved by the FDA for the treatment of dementia in PD patients and is the first agent approved for this indication.

Unfortunately, there have not been any head-to-head comparative studies on which to base preferences among these agents. For practical reasons, tacrine is usually least preferred because it requires laboratory monitoring for hepatotoxicity. However, two of these agents, donepezil and rivastigmine, have been tested in patients with dementia associated with PD or Lewy body disease. In a small crossover trial, 14 patients with PD and dementia were treated with donepezil and placebo.[31] There was some improvement in dementia, with no worsening of PD scores. This has been our clinical impression: that this drug is well tolerated from a motor point of view in patients with PD and dementia.

The much larger EXPRESS trial randomized 541 PD patients with dementia to receive either placebo or 3 mg to 12 mg of rivastigmine per day for 24 weeks.[32] Rivastigmine treatment was associated with significant, though moderate, improvements in dementia while where was a slight deterioration in those receiving placebo. However, there were significantly higher rates of nausea, vomiting, and tremor with rivastigmine. Of 433 patients who completed the double-blind trial, 334 entered and 273 completed an active treatment extension study.[33] At 48 weeks, the mean ADAS-cog score for the whole group improved by 2 points above baseline. Placebo patients switching to rivastigmine for the active treatment extension experienced a mean cognitive improvement similar to that of the original rivastigmine group during the double-blind trial. The adverse event profile was comparable to that seen in the double-blind trial.

In a separate study of rivastigmine in 120 patients with Lewy body disease and dementia, rivastigmine 3 mg to 12 mg daily was found to be tolerated and moderately effective. This same practice parameter states that rivastigmine should be considered (evidence level B) for treatment of the dementia of Lewy body disease.

It should be noted that a warning has been added to the package insert for galantamine because increased mortality observed in two 2-year, recent randomized, placebo-controlled trials in patients with mild-to-moderate cognitive impairment (MCI). The deaths were due to various causes that could be expected in an elderly population. About half of the deaths in patients receiving galantamine appeared to result from various vascular causes (myocardial infarction, stroke, and sudden death).

Control of agitated or disruptive behavior in demented PD patients is sometimes necessary. In such cases, management would be similar to that described below for psychosis in PD patients.

Psychosis
Psychosis in PD patients is of major concern since it is highly associated with nursing home placement

and increased mortality.[34] Approximately 20% to 40% of PD patients exhibit psychotic manifestations.[35,36] Psychosis tends to be more severe in patients with dementia or of advanced age. Visual hallucinations are particularly characteristic of psychosis in PD patients, while auditory and tactile hallucinations are rare. Delusions, usually paranoid in nature, are less common than hallucinations. In most cases, hallucinations are nonthreatening and recurrent but can be threatening or frightening in approximately 28% of patients.

Psychotic manifestations in PD patients usually result from an interaction between the underlying disease and its treatment. For example, excessive levodopa may cause hallucinations or psychosis in any patient with PD. In fact, all antiparkinsonian drugs have been implicated in various forms of psychosis. When given in combination, these medications appear to have a much higher propensity to produce confusional psychosis.

Management

The first step in management of drug-induced psychosis or hallucinations is to decrease or discontinue adjunctive therapy, including:

- Anticholinergics
- Amantadine
- Selegiline
- Dopamine agonists
- Benzodiazepines
- COMT inhibitors.

Decreasing the dose of levodopa should be attempted if psychosis continues. Unfortunately, these measures can worsen parkinsonism.

Cholinesterase inhibitors are currently considered first-line symptomatic therapy for mild psychosis in PD patients. Rivastigmine has recently gained approval from the FDA for the treatment of PD dementia. Small studies with donepezil,[37] rivastigmine,[38] and galantamine[39] have demonstrated their ability to relieve hallucinations. There are new prescribing warnings with galantamine concerning deaths in trials of patients who were studied for MCI.

In more severe cases, "atypical" neuroleptic agents at low doses are definitive therapy. Clozapine (Clozaril) is the most effective neuroleptic, and it does not aggravate the motor manifestations of PD.[40] However, because of the requirement of surveillance for agranulocytosis, clozapine is often considered a last resort. It is also associated with other bothersome side effects, including sialorrhea, weight gain, drowsiness, postural hypotension, and constipation. According to the most recent evidence-based practice parameter from the American Academy of Neurology, clozapine should be considered (evidence level B) and quetiapine (Seroquel) may be considered (evidence level C) for treatment of psychosis in PD patients.[41] Risperidone (Risperdal) and olanzapine (Zyprexa) will aggravate parkinsonism. According to this practice parameter, olanzapine should not be considered (evidence level B) for this indication. There is too little published experience with aripiprazole (Abilify) or ziprasidone (Geodon) in PD patients to assess their usefulness.

Although atypical neuroleptics can be effective in the management of psychosis in PD patients, the FDA recently issued an advisory regarding their use in the treatment of behavioral disorders in elderly patients with dementia. The FDA stated that clinical studies of these drugs in this population have shown a higher mortality rate associated with their use compared with patients receiving placebo.

Depression
Depression is the most common psychiatric complication of PD. Although estimates of the prevalence

of depression vary widely, an estimate of 40% is generally accepted when based on current diagnostic methods.[42] Depression in the setting of PD tends to remain in the mild to moderate range. Severe depression is unusual.[28] Whether depression is related to the loss of frontal dopaminergic projections or serotonin deficiency or is a psychological response to PD has not yet been resolved.[43] However, depression is clearly related to the "off" periods of levodopa response and lifts with improved control of motor symptoms.

Some of the physical manifestations of depression, such as weight loss, fatigue, insomnia, an inexpressive face, and slowness of movement, resemble those of PD. Therefore, it is sometimes difficult to determine if PD patients are depressed or when they are not. Physicians must simultaneously have a high index of suspicion for depression, and also be wary of over-diagnosing it in PD patients.

Management
_____

The response of depression to antiparkinsonian medication in PD patients is usually limited. Direct symptomatic therapy is almost always required. Therefore, depression in PD patients is treated in the same way are depression in other settings. Patients with PD and depression usually respond to treatment with conventional antidepressants. Sedating agents are useful for patients with sleep disorders, whereas those with apathetic depression may be helped by more stimulating agents. Mirtazapine is the only antidepressant reported to ameliorate, not aggravate, tremor[44] and also has sedating properties.

Anticholinergic and orthostatic adverse effects may limit the effectiveness or prevent the use of tricyclic agents (TCAs) in elderly patients. Of the available TCAs, trazodone has a lower anticholinergic potential and is often the better choice for these patients.

Before prescribing any antidepressant, it is important to consider any possible drug interactions with the patient's antiparkinsonian medication. All antidepressants are known to worsen rapid eye movement (REM)-sleep behavior disorder (RBD) (see below). Clinicians should be aware of this association.

The FDA has issued an advisory against concomitant use of selegiline and antidepressant medications because of the risk of "serotonin syndrome," which includes fever, restlessness, tremor, lethargy, and dysautonomia.[45] Although a serotonin syndrome is extremely rare, discontinuation of selegiline should be considered prior to taking antidepressant agents.

At least two studies have reported the successful use of electroconvulsive therapy (ECT) in severely depressed Parkinson patients.[46,47] Whether this is a true phenomenon is not yet clear, given the confounding variables in the studies. However, ECT may be the treatment of choice for severely depressed patients in whom medical management has failed or who have experienced intolerable side effects or confusion in response to an antidepressant.

Anxiety

Anxiety is characterized not only by feelings of apprehension and dread, but also autonomic manifestations such as hyperventilation, palpitation, dry mouth, and sweating. The incidence of anxiety in PD patients has been estimated to be 25%, but is higher in those who are also depressed.[48] Typically, anxiety develops after the diagnosis of PD, but may appear prior to motor symptoms. Anxiety symptoms often fluctuate along with motor symptoms in a levodopa dose-related fashion.[49,50]

Management

In patients in whom anxiety fluctuates with motor symptoms, treatment of the anxiety would be directed at eliminating or minimizing the fluctuations. Treatment of patients with nonfluctuating anxiety would be the same as in those in the general population and would involve selective serotonin reuptake inhibitors (SSRIs), other antidepressants, benzodiazepines, or buspirone. A recent, small study reported that citalopram treatment of depressed and anxious PD patients improved the depression as well as the anxiety.[51]

Apathy

Apathy is characterized by a loss of interest or motivation, resulting in reduced effort or initiative. It occurs more often in PD patients with depression, dementia, or bradyphrenia, but may exist independently. It is a poorly understood symptom, but one that results in a great deal of distress to the family unit. A small study by Isella and colleagues found that compared with normal controls, approximately 45% of PD patients exhibited apathy.[52] Like depression, many of the physical manifestations of apathy, such as flat affect, passivity, and lack of physical effort, can be mistaken for signs of PD. There is some evidence that apathy is distinct from depression,[53] and appears to correlate with cognitive impairment.[54]

Management

Although apathy may respond to dopaminergic medication in some PD patients, there currently is no consistently effective treatment for this symptom, although treatment with methylphenidate was found to be effective in a small case series.[55] A small pilot study in elderly male PD patients found that apathy was inversely correlated with plasma free testosterone levels, suggesting that testosterone replacement may be a potential treatment for apathy in this population.[56]

In my practice, I counsel the family and patient about this, indicating that it is not intentional and cannot be easily corrected. I recommend scheduled activities and encourage classes or programs that have been prepaid as an incentive for attendance. Students doing community service can be used to visit or engage the patient in meaningful activities. The most important aspect is to realize that the patient is not "lazy" but that there is a neurologic basis underlying this phenomenon.

■ Autonomic Disorders

Autonomic dysfunction, a common feature in PD, has been estimated to occur in 70% to 80% of all patients, with increasing frequency and severity with advancing disease. Many of the symptoms of autonomic dysfunction—particularly bladder, bowel, and sexual dysfunction—occur simultaneously resulting in a significant impact on the patient's quality of life.

Orthostatic Hypotension

When defined as a ≥20-mm Hg fall in systolic blood pressure (BP), orthostatic hypotension occurs in up to 60% of PD patients.[57] Advanced disease is correlated with an increased prevalence of orthostatic hypotension. It can be caused either by the disease itself or by the medications used to treat it. Any of the antiparkinsonian medications can cause or exacerbate hypotension, although the direct dopaminergic agonists are the most likely to do so. (When orthostatic hypotension is severe or is associated with other signs of autonomic dysfunction, such as disturbances of GI motility and urinary bladder function, the possibility of multisystem atrophy or Shy-Drager syndrome should be considered.) The use of diuretics, heat, and eating a large meal may all aggravate hypotension. The fall in BP may be large enough to result in syncope. However, hypotension may be subtler, resulting in feeling of nonspecific dizziness or lightheadedness, leg weakness, blurry vision, and can contribute to falls.[58]

Evaluation for orthostatic hypotension involves measuring BP in the lying and standing positions. In the upright position, the BP should be monitored for up to 10 minutes since the drop in BP may be gradual and delayed. The patient's current medication regimen should be reviewed for drugs that may be contributing to the hypotension, especially antihypertensives and diuretics.

Management

Management of orthostatic hypotension included both nonpharmacologic and pharmacologic measures[28]:

- Conservative measures:
  - Liberalize salt and fluid intake
  - Elevate head of bed
  - Sitting on edge of bed before standing
  - Compression stockings
  - Avoid heat, prolonged exercise
- Pharmacologic treatment:
  - Fludrocortisone (Florinef)
  - Midodrine (Pro-Amatine)
  - Pyridostigmine.

A number of pharmacologic agents can be used to increase BP. They include the mineralocorticoids, which increase sodium reabsorption in the kidney. The resultant exchange with potassium introduces the risk of hypokalemia, however. Thus prescribing or increasing a mineralocorticoid in patients with poor delivery of adequate sodium to the distal tubule is ineffective. In fact, a common mistake is the prescription of mineralocorticoids for patients on salt-restricted diets. Mineralocorticoids are likely to take several weeks to become effective. A suggested dosing schedule of fludrocortisone is 0.2 mg/day, increased to 0.4 mg/day as needed. Ankle edema and weight gain are expected side effects of fludrocortisone. In addition, patients should be watched for complications of the increased plasma volume, such as supine hypertension and symptoms of congestive heart failure

Midodrine, an α_1-adrenergic receptor agonist, is an appropriate option. Midodrine is a prodrug that, with its active metabolite desglymidodrine, produces increased vascular tone and an elevation in BP via activation of the α-adrenergic receptors of the arteriolar and venous vasculature. Administration of midodrine should start with 2.5 mg at breakfast and lunch followed by daily increases of 2.5-mg increments with a maximum 10 mg tid (every 4 hours upon rising, at midday, and late afternoon). Midodrine can be given at 3-hour intervals if needed but not more frequently and it should not be taken after 6 PM. The most noteworthy adverse events with midodrine include piloerection (goosebumps, tingling, and itching, especially of the scalp), urinary retention, and supine hypertension.

A recent report of the efficacy of pyridostigmine bromide in the treatment of orthostatic hypotension has allowed us one more treatment option for this troublesome syndrome. In this double-blind, randomized, 4-way cross-over study,[59] 58 patients with neurogenic orthostatic hypotension were given three active treatments (60 mg pyridostigmine; 60 mg pyridostigmine and 2.5 mg midodrine; 60 mg pyridostigmine and 5 mg of midodrine) or placebo in random order on successive days. The fall in standing diastolic BP was significantly reduced ($P = 0.02$) with treatment. Pairwise comparison showed significant reduction by pyridostigmine alone (BP fall of 27.6 mm Hg vs 34.0 mm Hg with placebo; $P = 0.04$) and pyridostigmine and 5 mg of midodrine hydrochloride (BP fall of 27.2 mm Hg vs 34.0 mm Hg with placebo; $P = 0.002$). The investigators concluded that pyridostigmine significantly improves standing BP in patients with orthostatic hypotension without worsening supine hypertension. The greatest effect is on diastolic BP, suggesting that the improvement is due to increased total peripheral resistance.

Combined use of any of these antihypotensive drugs with antihypertensive agents is often ineffective, resulting in exacerbation of both supine hypertension and orthostatic hypotension.[2]

Gastrointestinal Dysfunction

Nausea is a recognized, relatively common side effect of all dopaminergic agents. Taking carbidopa-levodopa with food is sometimes helpful. If this fails, addition of carbidopa in the form of a supplement is often effective in shunting levodopa into the brain. Should nausea remain a problem, a peripheral dopamine-blocking agent such as domperidone, which does not cross the blood-brain barrier, has been found to be extremely effective in reducing both nausea and postural hypotension. However, domperidone is not approved in the United States.

Gastrointestinal manifestations of autonomic dysfunction in PD patients may involve the entire length of the GI tract, and include dysphagia, sialorrhea, gastroparesis, and constipation.[60]

Dysphagia ultimately develops in a majority of PD patients and may result in aspiration. Patients should be monitored for coughing, gagging, or choking with meals, especially with liquids. Should any of these occur, formal evaluation of swallowing by a speech therapist is warranted. Management of dysphagia usually involves changes in dietary consistency and teaching the mechanical approach to swallowing.

Sialorrhea (drooling) is an embarrassing problem for many patients. In PD patients, sialorrhea is usually the result of decreased swallowing rather than excess production of saliva. Atropine-like drugs (eg, Sal-Tropine 0.4 mg bid) or anticholinergics are first-line treatment. Injection of botulinum toxin into the salivary glands can be helpful for severe drooling.[61,62]

Gastroparesis, which results in symptoms of post-prandial discomfort or bloating, early satiety, and nausea, is another common autonomic dysfunction in patients with PD. Gastroparesis in PD usually is a consequence of slowed gastric emptying time, which is even slower in patients receiving levodopa.[63] Management involves eating small, frequent meal, and discontinuation of medications (eg, anticholinergics) that impede gastric emptying. Although the peripheral dopamine antagonist domperidone has been shown to be effective,[64] this drug is not approved in the United States.

Constipation continues to be one of the most frequent autonomic-related complaints in PD patients at all stages of the disease. In addition to impaired motility, contributing factors include lack of dietary fiber, inadequate fluid intake, diminished physical activity, aging, and antiparkinsonian medications, including levodopa, dopamine agonists, anticholinergics, and amantadine. Anorectal dysfunction may also play a part.

Management of constipation includes nonpharmacologic as well as pharmacologic measures, such as[28]:

- Conservative measures:
  - Increase fluid intake
  - Increase dietary fiber
  - Increase activity level
- Pharmacologic treatment:
  - Discontinue anticholinergics
  - Bulk-forming agents
  - Stool softeners
  - Lubricants
  - Saline laxatives
  - Enemas.

A recipe that has proved effective for many patients; mix 1 cup bran, 1 cup applesauce, 1 cup prune juice. This mixture can be refrigerated, but any unused portion should be discarded after 1 week. Take 2 tbsp every morning, or mix 1 tbsp of each ingredient every morning as needed.

Genitourinary Dysfunction

Bladder dysfunction in PD patients may be related to overactive bladder with decreased capacity, manifested by frequency, urgency, nocturia, and incontinence, or expanded bladder capacity resulting in retention with decreased urinary stream, straining during voiding, and incomplete emptying. It can be difficult to distinguish between these two extremes without referral for cytometric studies. A hyperactive bladder can be quite distressing to patients with limited mobility.

The symptoms of hyperactive bladder can be managed with medications such as oxybutynin (Ditropan, Ditropan XL), tolterodine (Detrol, Detrol LA), or trospium chloride (Sanctura). Caution must be exercised as these agents have anticholinergic properties, possibly producing confusion and hallucinations in this susceptible population. For urinary retention, one can try terazosin (Hytrin), doxazosin (Cardura), or tamsulosin (Flomax).

Sexual dysfunction is also common in PD patients, and typically is characterized by difficulty with arousal and orgasmic function while interest in sexual activity is not usually affected.[65,66] While advanced age, depression, and severity of motor manifestations of PD contribute to sexual problems, autonomic dysfunction also plays a significant role.

Management involves sensitive but frank discussion of the sexual problems with patients and partner, including alternate methods of achieving sexual satisfaction or closeness with the partner.[67,68] Referral to counselors or specialists may be appropriate. Erectile dysfunction in male patients usually responds to sildenafil (Viagra), vardenafil (Levitra), or tadalafil

(Cialis). These medications should be prescribed cautiously since they may exacerbate postural hypotension. In some cases, yohimbine, papaverine, vacuum pumps, or penile implants may be appropriate.

Sweating/Thermoregulatory Dysfunction

Abnormal sympathetic skin responses, sweating, and thermoregulation related to autonomic dysfunction may also occur in patients PD. One pattern of abnormal sweating is characterized by a patchy loss of the ability to sweat. Another pattern is paroxysmal sweating that typically occurs at meal times or during the night. In the latter situation, the patient may awaken drenched in sweat and must change clothes.

Daytime sweating episodes may respond to SSRIs, while nighttime sweating may be controlled by clonidine 0.05 mg at bedtime.

■ Sleep Disorders

Sleep disorders have a major impact of the quality of life of PD patients and their families. They can occur at any stage of PD, but are common as the disease progresses. The prevalence of sleep disorders in PD patients ranges from 40% to 98%.[69,70] Typically, the earliest problem is sleep fragmentation. Other common sleep problems include difficulty initiating sleep, excessive daytime sleepiness (EDS), restless legs syndrome (RLS), RBD, sleep apnea, sleep walking, sleep talking nightmares, hallucinations, dyskinesias, nocturnal parkinsonism, or dementia-altered sleep-wake cycle.[71] Sleep problems may be a direct complication of PD or its treatment, or a consequence of nonmotor complications such as depression, nocturia, anxiety, or hallucinosis. A thorough assessment of sleep disorders should include complete medical and psychiatric histories, sleep history, and a 1- to 2-week sleep diary or Epworth Sleepiness Scale evaluation.[71] Polysomnography or actigraphy may also be useful. A recent review provides a comprehensive discussion the myriad sleep disorders seen in patients with PD, presents their diagnostic features, and gives recommendations on their management.[72]

Insomnia

Insomnia, caused either by difficulty falling asleep or frequent nocturnal awakening ("sleep fragmentation"), is a common complaint in PD patients. PD symptoms, such as tremor and akinesia with inability to turn in bed, nocturia, RLS, and hallucinations, can contribute to nocturnal awakenings.

Management of insomnia starts with identification and treatment of contributing factors and institution of good sleep hygiene measures, such as regular bedtimes, avoiding naps, exposure to sunlight during the day, sedentary evenings, and avoiding caffeine or large meals prior to sleep. Patients should also be advised to limit fluids to avoid nocturia. Care must then be given to bowel function to avoid constipation. Sedatives or sedating antidepressants can be employed for insomnia. The shorter-acting agents (zolpidem [Ambien]) can be given upon awakening in the night to restore sleep for the remainder of the night. If given at bedtime, however, there can be a wearing-off effect that may awaken the patient. Eszopiclone (Lunesta) is a recently approved agent.

If sleep is impaired because of resurgence of parkinsonian symptoms, a nighttime dose of dopaminergic medication can be helpful. This can take the form of long-acting levodopa, long-acting levodopa combined with a COMT inhibitor, or a dopamine agonist. However, in the patient with more advanced PD, this carries the risk of producing dyskinesias and interfering with sleep.

For nightmares and hallucinations, the use of an atypical neuroleptic, such as quetiapine or clozapine, can be considered. If depression accompanies the sleep disorder, any antidepressant can improve this situation. For the sedating action of antidepressants, trazodone or amitriptyline can be considered.

Excessive Daytime Sleepiness

EDS is common in PD patients and is related to disease severity, treatment, and the presence of other PD complications.[28] EDS is more prevalent in the more advanced stages of PD.[73] EDS is also associated with dopaminergic medication use, either dopamine agonists or levodopa.[74]

Reports of sudden-onset "sleep attacks" while driving in PD patients treated with dopamine agonists[75] raised serious concerns among patients, their families, and physicians. The occurrence of sleep attacks has been estimated to range from 6.6% of driving PD patients[76] to 20.8% of all PD patients.[77] Like EDS in general, sleep attacks are related to duration of PD,[78] and appear to be a nonspecific effect of all dopamine agonists,[79] as well as levodopa alone.[76]

Management of EDS begins by treating any contributing conditions and instituting good sleep hygiene as described above for insomnia. Reducing the dose, switching to an alternate dopaminergic agent, or eliminating potentially causative medications is the next step. Patients should be advised about the possibility of sudden sleep episodes that may result in motor vehicle accidents or other injury. Caffeine or other stimulants may provide symptomatic relief of EDS. While several early studies showed that the use of modafinal, a wake-promoting agent approved for use in narcolepsy, may be useful in patients with PD,[80-82] a more recent randomized, placcbo-controlled study found that modafinal failed to significantly improve EDS compared with placebo in PD patients as measured by the Epworth Sleepiness Score.[83]

REM-Sleep Behavior Disorder

RBD is characterized by loss of normal muscle atonia during REM sleep, which results in excessive motor activity while dreaming. Affected individuals may thrash, kick, punch, or yell out phrases such as "Get away from me!" while dreaming. They generally have no recollection of this behavior when they awake in the morning, although if awakened during an episode, they may describe dreams about physical conflict or being chased. The best clinical diagnostic tool is to ask the spouse/bed partner: "Does your spouse (or significant other) act out their dreams?"

RBD in PD patients is very responsive to clonazepam 0.5 to 2 mg at bedtime.

Restless Legs Syndrome

RLS is characterized by an irresistible urge of move the limbs. Onset is usually unilateral in 40% to 50% of cases, and the arms may be affected in 25% to 50% of patients.[28] It generally occurs when the legs are at rest (sitting or lying down). Although this is an idiopathic disorder distinct from PD, it is often associated with PD. It may be a challenge to differentiate restless legs from akathisia (see below). The symptoms of RLS, aching, burning, and cramping, can be very distressing and may contribute to insomnia by delaying the onset of sleep. Walking relieves the symptoms. Approximately 20% of PD patients have symptoms consistent with RLS and in >70%, the onset of PD preceded or occurred concomitantly with the development of RLS.[84]

RLS generally is responsive to dopaminergic medication, particularly dopamine agonists. Low doses of pramipexole (0.125 to 0.5 mg) or ropinirole (0.25 to 1 mg) at bedtime are usually effective.[28] Other possibly effective agents include gabapentin, clonazepam, and opiates.

- **Sensory Disorders**

Akathisia is a sensation of restlessness. It is experienced as a feeling of relentless and overwhelming need to move or an inability to remain still. Movement does not provide relief. Patients may also feel anxiety, panic, and irritability. Akathisia may be exhibit this inner sense of restlessness by pacing, body rocking, leg swinging, or toe tapping. Akathisia can occur at any time of the day. Most patients taking levodopa do not note a relationship between akathisia and the timing of their medication, although some experience a fluctuating phenomenon.[28]

In patients with fluctuating akathisia, adjustment of their PD medications may be helpful. In other cases, symptomatic treatment may be attempted with agents such as β-blockers, anticholinergics, amantadine, clonidine, mirtazapine, or benzodiazepines. However, treatment response of akathisia is usually modest at best.[28]

Olfactory dysfunction, a decrease or loss of the olfactory sense, is common in PD patients and usually precedes the onset of motor symptoms. Unfortunately, no effective treatment is known.

- **Weight Loss**

As in patients with many chronic diseases, those with PD often lose weight over time. A variety of factors for weight loss in PD patients have been proposed, including a hypermetabolic state resulting from the increase muscular effort for rigidity and involuntary movements, the nauseating effects of levodopa, malabsorption, dysphagia, the high prevalence of depression, and the low-protein (protein redistribution) diet. However, there is no consensus about the mechanisms of weight loss.

Weight loss in PD patients may be reversed by successful medical treatment of PD.[28] High-calorie, high-protein diets and dietary supplements also can help. Several recent studies have reported that weight loss can be reversed by pallidotomy or subthalamic nucleus deep brain stimulation.[85,86]

■ Driving

Driving can become problematic in patients with PD for several reasons. Reaction times may be slowed and patients may have impaired visuospatial abilities. Those with more advanced disease may have impaired cognition and judgment and, as discussed above, some patients may experience "sleep attacks."

Physicians are sometimes asked for an opinion regarding an individual patient's competence to drive an automobile. This can present a sensitive situation since the request for the physician's opinion often follows a period of emotional discussions among relatives. For the patient, it may be an issue of personal independence and self-image.

Evaluation of a patient's ability to drive requires a combined evaluation of motor and nonmotor symptoms and signs, especially akinesia and dementia. Although a purely clinical assessment may overestimate a patient's driving abilities, two recent comparative studies identified significant correlations between several clinical findings and driving ability. One study in 18 PD patients and 18 healthy controls examined the correlation between neuropsychological test performance and driving simulator behavior.[87] The results in PD patients suggest that impaired executive function, such as working memory, planning, and set shifting, are associated with reduced tactical level driving performance, such as speed adaptation and complex curve navigation. Impaired information processing, visual attention and visual perception were associated with reduced driving performance, such as reacting to road obstacles and maintaining constant lane position.

In a second study, 25 PD patients and 21 age-matched controls, all regular drivers, underwent neurological evaluation and assessment of cognitive, visual, and motor function and a standardized, on-road driving assessment.[88] The objective of this study was to assess the ability of individual tests to predict pass/fail driving outcomes. Three tests from the larger battery (Purdue Pegboard test for motor performance, Pelli-Robson test for contrast sensitivity, and the verbal version of Symbol Digit Modalities test for cognitive function) predicted passes with relatively high sensitivity (PD, 72.7%; controls, 93.8%; both combined, 85.2%); and moderate specificity (PD, 64.3%; controls, 60.0%; both combined. 63.2%). Adding time since diagnosis for the PD group increased sensitivity to 90.9% and specificity to 71.4%.

These clinical assessments may be useful, expecially useful when on-road assessments are not feasible. In most cases, however, a formal driving assessment performed by an occupational therapy specialist in a driving simulator or on the road provides a more reliable evaluation. In such cases, patients may be more apt to accept the results since they carry the aura of being an independent, third-party decision.

REFERENCES

1. Jankovic J. Motor fluctuations and dyskinesias in Parkinson's disease: clinical manifestations. *Mov Disord.* 2005;20(suppl): S11-S16. Published online: April 8, 2005; DOI: 10.1002/mds.20458.

2. Waters CH. Managing the late complications of Parkinson's disease. *Neurology.* 1997;49(suppl 1):S49-S57.

3. Olanow CW, Agid Y, Mizuno Y, et al. Levodopa in the treatment of Parkinson's disease: current controversies. *Mov Disord.* 2004;19:997-1005.

4. Metman LV, Konitsiotis S, Chase TN. Pathophysiology of motor response complications in Parkinson's disease: hypotheses on the why, where, and what. *Mov Disord.* 2000;15:3-8.

5. Silver GA, Vuong K, Jankovic J. Young-onset versus late-onset Parkinson's disease: Clinical features and disease progression. *Mov Disord.* 2004;19(suppl 9):S264.

6. Ahlskog JE, Muenter MD. Frequency of levodopa-related dyskinesias and motor fluctuations as estimated from the cumulative literature. *Mov Disord.* 2001;16:448-458.

7. Parkinson Study Group. Impact of deprenyl and tocopherol treatment on Parkinson's disease in DATATOP patients requiring levodopa. *Ann Neurol.* 1996;39:37-45.

8. Block G, Liss C, Reines S, Irr J, Nibbelink D. Comparison of immediate-release and controlled release carbidopa/levodopa in Parkinson's disease. A multicenter 5-year study. The CR First Study group. *Eur Neurol.* 1997;37:23-27.

9. Nutt JG, Carter JH, Van Houten L, Woodward WR. Short- and long-duration responses to levodopa during the first year of levodopa therapy. *Ann Neurol.* 1997;42:349-355.

10. Fahn S, Oakes D, Shoulson I, et al; Parkinson Study Group. Levodopa and the progression of Parkinson's disease. *N Engl J Med.* 2004;351:2498-2508.

11. Waters C. Other pharmacologic treatments for motor complications and dyskinesias. *Mov Disord.* 2005;20(suppl):S38-S44. Published online April 8, 2005; DOI: 10/1002/mds.20462.

12. Pahwa R, Factor SA, Lyons KE, et al; Quality Standards Subcommittee of the American Academy of Neurology. Practice Parameter: treatment of Parkinson disease with motor fluctuations and dyskinesia (an evidence-based review): report of the Quality Standards Subcommittee of the American Academy of Neurology. *Neurology.* 2006;66:983-995.

13. Ondo W, Hunter C, Almaguer M, Jankovic J. A novel sublingual apomorphine treatment for patients with fluctuating Parkinson's disease. *Mov Disord.* 1999;14:664-668.

14. Priano L, Albani G, Calderoni S, et al. Controlled-release transdermal apomorphine treatment for motor fluctuations in Parkinson's disease. *Neurol Sci.* 2002;23(suppl 2):S99-S100.

9

15. Hutton JT, Metman LV, Thomas NC, et al. Transdermal dopaminergic D2 receptor agonist therapy in Parkinson's disease with N-0923 TDS: a double-blind, placebo-controlled study. *Mov Disord.* 2001;16:459-463.

16. Metman LV, Gillespie M, Farmer C, et al. Continuous transdermal dopaminergic stimulation in advanced Parkinson's disease. *Clin Neuropharmacol.* 2001;24:163-169.

17. Giladi N, Gurevich T, Shabtai H, Paleacu D, Simon ES. The effect of botulinum toxin injections to the calf muscles on freezing of gait in parkinsonism: a pilot study. *J Neurol* 2001;248:572-576.

18. Vidailhet M, Bonnet AM, Marconi N, Durif F, Agid Y. The phenomenology of L-dopa-induced dyskinesias in Parkinson's disease. *Mov Disord.* 1999;14(suppl 1):13-18.

19. Marconi R, Lefebvre-Caparros D, Bonnet AM, Vidailhet M, Dubois B, Agid Y. Levodopa-induced dyskinesia in Parkinson's disease: phenomenology and pathophysiology. *Mov Disord.* 1994;9:2-12.

20. Metman LV, Del Dotto P, LePoole K, Konitsiotis S, Fang J, Chase TN. Amantadine for levodopa-induced dyskinesias in Parkinson's disease. A 1-year follow-up study. *Arch Neurol.* 1999;56:1383-1386.

21. Snow BJ, Macdonald L, Mcauley D, Wallis W. The effect of amantadine on levodopa-induced dyskinesias in Parkinson's disease: a double-blind, placebo-controlled study. *Clin Neuropharmacol.* 2000;23:82-85.

22. Thomas A, Iacono D, Luciano AL, Armellino K, Di Iorio A, Onofrj M. Duration of amantadine benefit in dyskinesia of severe Parkinson's disease. *J Neurol Neurosurg Psychiatry.* 2004;75:141-143.

23. Durif F, Vidailhet M, Assal F, Poche C, Bonnet AM, Agid Y. Low-dose clozapine improves dyskinesias in Parkinson's disease. *Neurology.* 1997;48:658-662.

24. Durif F, Debilly B, Galitzky M, et al. Clozapine improves dyskinesias in Parkinson's disease: a double-blind, placebo-controlled study. *Neurology.* 2004;62:381-388.

25. Carpentier AF, Bonnet AM, Vidailhet M, Agid Y. Improvement of levodopa-induced dyskinesia by propranolol in Parkinson's disease. *Neurology.* 1996;46:1548-1551.

26. Lhermitte F, Agid Y, Signoret JL. Onset and end-of-dose levodopa-induced dyskinesias. *Arch Neurol.* 1978;35:261-263.

27. Shulman LM, Taback RL, Bean J, Weiner WJ. Comorbidity of the nonmotor symptoms of Parkinson's disease. *Mov Disord.* 2001;16:507-510.

28. Riley D. Non-motor manifestations of Parkinson's disease. In: *Course Syllabus: Practical Management of Motor Complications in Parkinson's Disease.* The Movement Disorder Society; May 22, 2004.

29. Marder K, Jacobs DM. Dementia. In: Factor S, Weiner WJ, eds. *Parkinson's Disease: Diagnosis and Clinical Management.* New York, NY: Demos; 2002:125-135.

30. Foltynie T, Brayne CE, Robbins TW, Barker RA. The cognitive ability of an incident cohort of Parkinson's patients in the UK. The CamPaIGN study. *Brain.* 2004;127:550-560.

31. Aarsland D, Larsen JP, Janvin C. Donepezil treatment in Parkinson's disease with dementia: a double-blind, placebo-controlled crossover study. *Neurology.* 2001;56(suppl 3):A128. Abstract.

32. Emre M, Aarsland D, Albanese A, et al. Rivastigmine for dementia associated with Parkinson's disease. *N Engl J Med.* 2004;351:2509-2518.

33. Poewe W, Wolters E, Emre M, et al; EXPRESS Investigators. Long-term benefits of rivastigmine in dementia associated with Parkinson's disease: an active treatment extension study. *Mov Disord.* 2006;21:456-461.

34. Factor SA, Feustel PJ, Friedman JH, et al; Parkinson Study group. Longitudinal outcome of Parkinson's disease patients with psychosis. *Neurology.* 2003;60:1756-1761.

35. Factor SA, Molho ES, Podskalny GD, Brown D. Parkinson's disease: drug-induced psychiatric states. *Adv Neurol.* 1995; 65:115-138.

9

36. Fenelon G, Mahieux F, Huon R, Ziegler M. Hallucinations in Parkinson's disease: prevalence, phenomenology and risk factors. *Brain.* 2000;123:733-745.

37. Fabbrini G, Barbanti P, Aurilia C, Pauletti C, Lenzi GL, Meco G. Donepezil in the treatmetn of hallucatinations and delusions in Parkinson's disease. *Neurol Sci.* 2002;23:41-43.

38. Bullock R, Cameron A. Rivastigmine for the treatment of dementia and visual hallucinations in Parkinson's disease. *Curr Med Res Opin.* 2002;18:258-264.

39. Aarsland D, Hutchinson M, Larsen JP. Cognitive, psychiatric and motor response to galantamine in Parkinson's disease with dementia. *Int J Geriatr Psychiatry.* 2003;18:937-941.

40. The Parkinson Study Group. Low-dose clozapine for the treatment of drug-induced psychosis in Parkinson's disease. *N Engl J Med.* 1999;340:757-763.

41. Miyasaki JM, Shannon K, Voon V, et al; Quality Standards Subcommittee of the American Academy of Neurology. Practice Parameter: evaluation and treatment of depression, psychosis, and dementia in Parkinson disease (an evidence-based review): report of the Quality Standards Subcommittee of the American Academy of Neurology. *Neurology.* 2006;66:996-1002.

42. Mayberg HS, Solomon DH. Depression in Parkinson's disease: a biochemical and organic viewpoint. *Adv Neurol.* 1995;65:49-60.

43. Poewe W, Luginger E. Depression in Parkinson's disease: impediments to recognition and treatment options. *Neurology.* 1999;52(suppl 3):S2-S6.

44. Pact V, Giduz T. Mirtazapine treats resting tremor, essential tremor, and levodopa-induced dyskinesias. *Neurology.* 1999;53:1154.

45. Richard IH, Kurlan R, Tanner C, et al. Serotonin syndrome and the combined use of deprenyl and an antidepressant in Parkinson's disease. Parkinson Study Group. *Neurology.* 1997;48:1070-1077.

46. Stern MB. Electroconvulsive therapy in untreated Parkinson's disease. *Mov Disord.* 1991;6:265.

47. Faber R, Trimble MR. Electroconvulsive therapy in Parkinson's disease and other movement disorders. *Mov Disord.* 1991;6:293-303.

48. Menza MA, Robertson-Hoffman DE, Bonapace AS. Parkinson's disease and anxiety: comorbidity with depression. *Biol Psychiatry.* 1993;34:465-470.

49. Maricle RA, Nutt JG, Valentine RJ, Carter JH. Dose-response relationship of levodopa with mood and anxiety in fluctuating Parkinson's disease: a double-blind, placebo controlled study. *Neurology.* 1995;45:1757-1760.

50. Richard IH, Frank S, McDermott MP, et al. The ups and downs of Parkinson's disease: a prospective study of mood and anxiety. *Cogn Behav Neurol.* 2004;17:201-207.

51. Menza MA, Marin H, Kaufman K, Mark M, Lauritano M. Citalopram treatment of depression in Parkinson's disease: the impact on anxiety, disability and cognition. *J Neuropsychiatry Clin Neurosci.* 2004;16:315-319.

52. Isella V, Melzi P, Grimaldi M, et al. Clinical, neuropsychological, and morphometric correlates of apathy in Parkinson's disease. *Mov Disord.* 2002;17:366-371.

53. Levy ML, Cummings JL, Fairbanks LA, et al. Apathy is not depression. *J Neuropsychiatry Clin Neurosci.* 1998;10:314-319.

54. Pluck GC, Brown RG. Apathy in Parkinson's disease. *J Neurol Neurosurg Psychiatry.* 2002;73:636-642.

55. Chatterjee A, Fahn S. Methylphenidate treats apathy in Parkinson's disease. *J Neuropsychiatry Clin Neurosci.* 2002; 14:461-462.

56. Ready RE, Friedman J, Grace J, Fernandez H. Testosterone deficiency and apathy in Parkinson's disease: a pilot study. *J Neurol Neurosurg Psychiatry.* 2004;75:1323-1326.

9

57. Senard JM, Rai S, Lapeyre-Mestre M, et al. Prevalence of orthostatic hypotension in Parkinson's disease. *J Neurol Neurosurg Psychiatry.* 1997;63:584-589.

58. Hillen ME, Wagner ML, Sage JI. "Subclinical" orthostatic hypotension is associated with dizziness in elderly patients with Parkinson's disease. *Arch Phys Med Rehabil.* 1996; 77:710-712.

59. Singer W, Sandroni P, Opfer-Gehrking TL, et al. Pyridostigmine treatment trial in neurogenic orthostatic hypotension. *Arch Neurol.* 2006;63:513-518.

60. Pfeiffer RF. Gastrointestinal dysfunction in Parkinson's disease. *Lancet Neurol.* 2003;2:107-116.

61. Mancini F, Zangaglia R, Cristina S, et al. Double-blind, placebo-controlled study to evaluate the efficacy and safety of botulinum toxin type A in the treatment of drooling in parkinsonism. *Mov Disord.* 2003;18:685-688.

62. Ondo WG, Hunter C, Moore W. A double-blind placebo-controlled trial of botulinum toxin B for sialorrhea in Parkinson's disease. *Neurology.* 2004;62:37-40.

63. Hardoff R, Sula M, Tamir A, et al. Gastric emptying time and gastric motility in patients with Parkinson's disease. *Mov Disord.* 2001;16:1041-1047.

64. Jost WH. Gastrointestinal motility problems in patients with Parkinson's disease. Effects of antiparkinsonian treatment and guidelines for management. *Drugs Aging.* 1997;10:249-258.

65. Bronner G, Royter V, Korczyn AF, Giladi N. Sexual dysfunction in Parkinson's disease. *J Sex Marital Ther.* 2004;30: 95-105.

66. Yu M, Roane DM, Miner CR, Fleming M, Rogers JD. Dimensions of sexual dysfunction in Parkinson's disease. *Am J Geriatr Psychiatry.* 2004;12:221-226.

67. Waters CH, Smolowitz J. Impaired sexual function. In: Ebadi M, Pfeiffer RF, eds. *Parkinson's Disease.* Boca Raton, Fla: CRC Press LLC; 2005:287-294.

68. Waters CH, Smolowitz L. Hyposexual function. In: Pfeiffer RF, Bodis-Wollner I, eds. *Parkinson's Disease and Nonmotor Dysfunction*. Totowa, NJ: Humana Press; 2005.

69. Tandberg E, Larsen JP, Karlsen K. A community-based study of sleep disorders in patients with Parkinson's disease. *Mov Disord.* 1998;13:895-899.

70. Kumar S, Bhatia M, Behari M. Sleep disorders in Parkinson's disease. *Mov Disord.* 2002;17:775-781.

71. Thorpy MJ, Sleep disorders in Parkinson's disease. *Clin Cornerstone.* 2004;6(suppl 1A):S7-S15.

72. Adler CH, Thorpy MJ. Sleep issues in Parkinson's disease. *Neurology.* 2005;64(suppl 3):S12-S20.

73. Kumar S, Bhatia M, Behari M. Excessive daytime sleepiness in Parkinson's disease as assessed by Epworth Sleepiness Scale (ESS). *Sleep Med.* 2003;4:339-342.

74. Garcia-Borreguero D, Schwarz C, Larrosa O, de la Llave Y, Garcia de Yebenes J. L-dopa-induced excessive daytime sleepiness in PD: a placebo-controlled case with MSLT assessment. *Neurology.* 2003;61:1008-1010.

75. Frucht S, Rogers JD, Greene PE, Gordon MF, Fahn S. Falling asleep at the wheel: motor vehicle mishaps in persons taking pramipexole and ropinirole. *Neurology.* 1999;52:1908-1910.

76. Homann CN, Wenzel K, Suppan K, et al. Sleep attacks in patients taking dopamine agonists: review. *BMJ.* 2002;324:1483-1487.

77. Brodsky MA, Godbold J, Roth T, Olanow CW. Sleepiness in Parkinson's disease: a controlled study. *Mov Disord.* 2003;18:668-672.

78. Paus S, Brecht HM, Koster J, Seeger G, Klockgether T, Wullner U. Sleep attacks, daytime sleepiness, and dopamine agonists in Parkinson's disease. *Mov Disord.* 2003;18:1569-1570.

79. Roth T. Rye DB, Borchert LD, et al. Assessment of sleepiness and unintended sleep in Parkinson's disease patients taking dopamine agonists. *Sleep Med.* 2003;4:275-280.

80. Nieves AV, Lang AE. Treatment of excessive daytime sleepiness in patients with Parkinson's disease with modafinil. *Clin Neuropharmacol.* 2002;25:111-114.

81. Adler CH, Caviness JN, Hentz JG, Lind M, Tiede J. Randomized trial of modafinal for treating subjective daytime sleepiness in patients with Parkinson's disease. *Mov Disord.* 2003;18:287-293.

82. Hogl B, Saletu M, Branauer E, et al. Modafinil for the treatment of daytime sleepiness in Parkinson's disease: a double-blind, randomized, crossover, placebo-controlled polygraphic trial. *Sleep.* 2002;25:905-909.

83. Ondo WG, Fayle R, Atassi F, Jankovic J. Modafinil for daytime somnolence in Parkinson's disease: double blind, placebo controlled parallel trial. *J Neurol Neurosurg Psychiatry.* 2005;76:1636-1639.

84. Ondo WG, Vuong KD, Jankovic J. Exploring the relationship between Parkinson's disease and restless legs syndrome. *Arch Neurol.* 2002;59:421-424.

85. Ondo WG, Ben-Aire L, Jankovic J, Lai E, Contant C, Grossman R. Weight gain following unilateral pallidotomy in Parkinson's disease. *Acta Neurol Scand.* 2000;101:79-84.

86. Barichella M, Marczewska AM, Mariani C, Landi A, Vairo A, Pezzoli G. Body weight gain rate in patients with Parkinson's disease and deep brain stimulation. *Mov Disord.* 2003;18:1337-1340.

87. Stolwyk RJ, Charlton JL, Triggs TJ, Iansek R, Bradshaw JL. Neuropsychological function and driving ability in people with Parkinson's disease. *J Clin Exp Neuropsychol.* 2006;28:898-913.

88. Worringham CJ, Wood JM, Kerr GK, Silburn PA. Predictors of driving assessment outcome in Parkinson's disease. *Mov Disord.* 2006;21:230-235.

10 Nonpharmacologic Management of Parkinson's Disease

Nonpharmacologic therapy, especially psychological support, is of incalculable value from diagnosis throughout the course of Parkinson's disease (PD).[1] Patients derive benefit from the knowledge that the disease is an area of active research and that increasingly effective medications and other interventions are on the horizon. Patients with careers and young families need realistic prognostic information, which often relieves excessive fears of early disability.

A suggested timetable for discussion of the disease and its implications for patients' future quality of life is seen in **Table 10.1**. Heritability is not discussed unless the patient has a positive family history since the hereditary pattern remains unclear and not amenable to genetic counseling.

Recommendation that patients join a support group is put off until initial stress of the diagnosis has passed and they are able to cope with seeing patients in more advanced stages of the disease. The timing of additional, more distressing topics, such as the probability of dementia, impotence, and incontinence, is probably best left to the patient.

The comprehensive management of PD patients is a team effort involving a variety of therapeutic interventions and therapists, including the[2]:

- Primary physician
- Neurologist
- Family members
- Physical, occupational, speech therapists.

TABLE 10.1 — Topics for Discussion Early in the Course of Parkinson's Disease	
Approximate Timing	**Topic**
At diagnosis	• Outline general nature of PD and its treatability
Postdiagnosis	
1-2 months	• Explain prognosis of typical case • Outline ongoing research related to prophylaxis and treatment • Recommend lay literature • Recommend joining national support societies • Follow-up rereading, national support societies

8 months	• Educate regarding treatment complications to be aware of:
	  – Dose-related wearing-off
	  – Dyskinesia
	  – Mental difficulty

2 years	• Recommend joining local support group • Recommend regular exercise schedule, if patient is sedentary
Abbreviation: PD, Parkinson's disease.	
Adapted from: Kurlan R, ed. *Treatment of Movement Disorders*. Philadelphia, Pa: JB Lippincott Co; 1995:1-56.	

Although the diagnosis and management plan of PD and related movement disorders are largely handled by neurologists, family or primary physicians are frequently the first to be consulted by patients with early parkinsonian signs and symptoms. They are often the first to suspect the diagnosis and to refer patients to specialists and are likely to provide coordination of therapy thereafter.

Family members are regularly involved in care, and as disability progresses, often become the primary caregivers, supported by home health care nursing, physicians, and specialized therapists.

The primary physician, with the assistance of an occupational therapist, must assess limitations of the patient's daily activities as they occur. Activities to be evaluated regularly include:

- Grooming
- Dressing
- Walking
- Eating
- Washing dishes
- Playing cards
- Writing letters
- Reading the newspaper
- Housecleaning
- Making beds
- Cooking meals
- Gardening
- Driving.

Environmental Modifications

The first level of adaptation to PD centers around the patient's environment, which should be evaluated during a home visit by an occupational therapist. Patient and family should be questioned about:

- Doorsills
- Scatter rugs
- Furniture in high-traffic areas of the house
- Faucet and door handles that are difficult to use
- Other structural impediments to daily living.

Simple adaptations of these environmental barriers can be helpful in fostering an active existence. Some specific modifications include:

- A bed low enough to allow the patient to rise easily
- A chair with arm rests and a firm seat to facilitate dressing
- A urinal or commode near the bed for nighttime use
- If stiffness is a problem, a bed cradle made from a sturdy cardboard box will keep bedclothes from entangling feet and lower legs when patient turns in bed
- A trapeze over head of the bed or a cord attached to the frame may help in changing positions or rising
- Button fasteners, zipper extensions, elastic shoe laces.

In the bathroom, the patient's life can be made simpler by:
- A raised toilet seat and a grab bar on the adjacent wall
- A toothpaste tube squeezer and a large-handled toothbrush
- An electric razor
- Tub and shower seats and grab bars
- Grooming aids in the shower, including a suction brush, soap on a rope, a sponge on a long handle.

In the kitchen, a number of adaptations can facilitate patients' daily life, including:
- Utensils with large handles and knives that cut with rocking motion
- Combination utensils, such as combined fork and spoon
- Easy-hold cups, flexible plastic straws, and non-skid plates
- Jar-lid openers
- Wooden reachers.

A few general, practical aids available from occupational therapists can also be recommended to help in the activities of daily living, including:

- A push-button telephone adapter with large keys to prevent misdialing
- Risers under the rear legs of straight-back chairs to help patient stand up (usually preferable to spring chairs or devices with wheels, which may be more dangerous than helpful)
- A book holder to help stabilize pages.

Driving

Driving may be an integral part of the Parkinson patient's life and, therefore, may be a significant indication of his or her independence. Considerations in assessing driving ability should include:

- Judgment
- Mental status
- Reaction speed.

Side effects of medication must also be considered in this context. The tendency to freeze can be fatal. Since the decision regarding driving is always difficult, the most objective approach is to have the patient take an approved driver instruction course or retake the state driver's license test.

Patient Education

Many patient education resources are available from the various foundations and associations devoted to PD (**Table 10.2**). Physicians recommending these materials should be familiar with their contents, however, since recommendation implies endorsement.

TABLE 10.2 — Parkinson's Disease Foundations

American Parkinson's Disease Association, Inc.
1250 Hylan Boulevard, Suite 4B
Staten Island, NY 10305
(718) 981-8001
(800) 223-2732
Website: www.apdaparkinson.org

The Michael J. Fox Foundation
  for Parkinson's Research
P.O. Box 4777 Grand Central Station
New York, NY 10163
(800) 708-7644
Website: www.michaeljfox.org

National Parkinson Disease Association
1501 NW 9th Ave, Bob Hope Road
Miami, FL 33136-1494
(305) 243-6666
(800) 243-5595
Website: www.parkinson.org

Parkinson Action Network
1025 Vermont Ave. NW, Suite 1120
(202) 638-4101
(800) 850-4726
Website: www. parkinsonsaction.org

Parkinson's Disease Foundation, Inc.
1359 Broadway, Suite 1509
New York, NY 10018
(212) 923-4700
(800) 457-6676
Website: www.pdf.org

Parkinson Society Canada
4211 Yonge Street, Suite 316
Toronto, ON M2P 2A9
Canada
(416) 227-9700
(800) 565-3000
Website: www.parkinson.ca

Continued

European Parkinson Disease Association
4 Golding Road
Seven Oaks
Kent, UK TN13 3NJ
Website: www.epda.eu.com

Physical Therapy

Walking 1 mile a day is often considered a reasonable goal, although many patients can walk much farther than that. Swimming is often recommended, especially for patients who swam earlier in life. It may also be useful for patients with asymmetrical disease, since it forces them to use the more affected side in order to swim in a straight line.

Patients who play golf, tennis, or racquetball or those who hike, bicycle, or jog should be encouraged to continue these activities on a regular basis. Others benefit from ballroom or square dancing. Some simple exercises that can be adapted for home use are illustrated in **Figure 10**.1.

As PD advances, most patients will benefit from formal physical therapy, which should be based on a needs assessment and specific goals. Prescribed exercises may improve the shuffling gait, stooped posture, and postural instability.

■ Tremor, Rigidity, Bradykinesia

Although these cardinal features of PD cannot be eliminated by nonpharmacologic approaches, their impact on patients' functional status can often be alleviated with physical and occupational therapy. In addition to the exercises described in **Figure 10**.1, a few additional simple ones may relieve functional disability due to rigidity and bradykinesia (**Table 10**.3).

Physical therapy may also help patients with rigidity and akinesia and disordered movement patterns. The approach involves practicing simple movements,

FIGURE 10.1 — Selected Exercises With Verbal Cues for the Parkinson's Disease Patient

Back Thigh Stretches

This exercise is designed to reduce tightness and cramping in the back thigh muscles.

Position

Lie on your back with your knees bent. Arms are stretched above your head.

Action

- Raise your right knee.
- Stretch your heel toward the ceiling.
- Point your toes toward your nose.
- Bend your right knee and place it back at the start position.
- Repeat, raising the right knee.
- Stretch your heel toward the ceiling.
- Point your toes toward your nose.
- Do ten stretches, alternating legs.

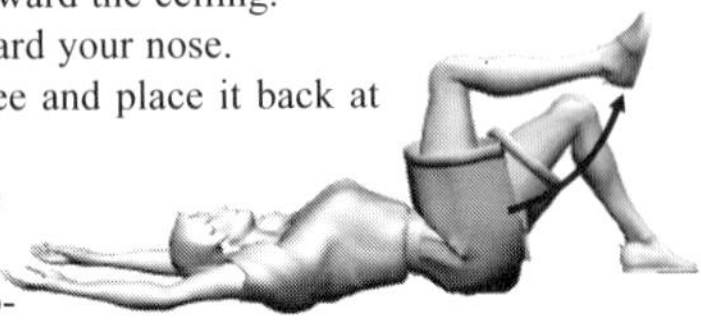

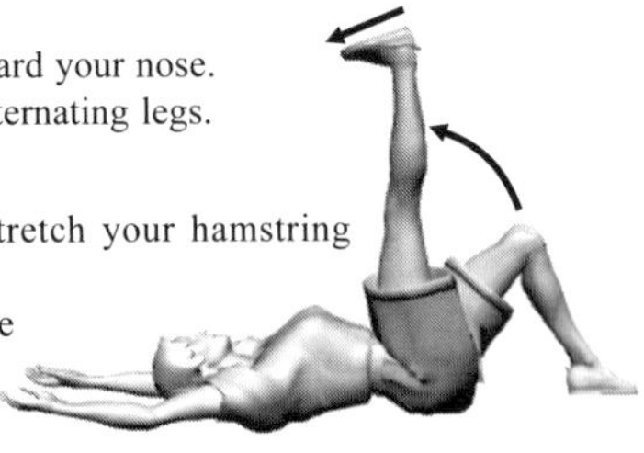

Verbal Cues

"Try ten to really stretch your hamstring muscles."

"One... Right knee up, heel toward the ceiling, toes point to nose and down."

"Two... Left knee up, heel up, toes point to nose and down."

"Three... Right up, heel up, toes point, watch your leg, and down."

"Four... Left up, stretch your leg, point your toes, down."

"Five... Right, feel the stretch. Really stretch! Down."

"Six... Left, count along. You can do it! Good."

"Seven... Right knee up, heel up, toes point, and relax."

"Eight... Left, lift, now you have got it! Fine, lower."

"Nine... Right, raise that leg. Stretch the thigh and ankle, lower."

"Ten... Left, make this last one really count. Good! And, rest."

Continued

High-Step Marching

Marching while walking is designed to challenge you to lift your feet with every step and also loosens the hips.

Action

Bring your toes and knee up with every step you take. March as you walk.

Verbal Cues

"March with the music."
"March right, march left, and right, and left, lift toes, lift high. Good. Right, march left, march right, march left." "Continue with the music and lift, and right, and left, right, left, right, left, right, left, return to your starting point and relax. Good."

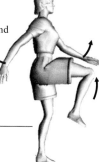

Arm X's and Y's

This exercise is helpful for your deep breathing and posture.

Position

Lie on your back. Your legs are straight, hands crossed and touching your upper thighs.

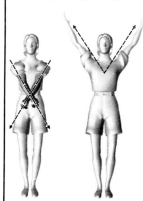

Action

- Spread your hands as you inhale and raise the arms over your head up and out to make a V.
- Make fists and exhale as you lower your arms across your hips making an X.
- Rest and repeat 10 times.
- At another time; sit in a straight chair with your wrists crossed on top of your knees.
- Perform this movement as above from the seated position.

- For more exertion, small hand weights may be used to increase your strength.

Verbal Cues

"Loosen your shoulders as well as improve your breathing. Count loudly for ten."

Continued

"One… Up, open your hands, inhale as you stretch up and out and make a V."

"Two… Down, exhale, closing your fists as you lower arms crossed to make an X."

"Three… Up, inhale, open hands, stretch up and out, over your head."

"Four… Down, exhale, make a fist, lower your arms down and across hips."

"Five… Way up now! Inhale deeply. Are you making a Y?"

"Six… Cross down, breathe all the way out, form an X."

"Seven… Up, make a V. Look at your hands as you stretch further. Good!"

"Eight… Down, cross the arms as you look down."

"Nine… Inhale and up. Look and count."

"Ten… Breathe out, and down. Fine and rest."

Shift, Lift, and Step

*This exercise is helpful when you
need extra momentum to get unglued.*

Position

Stand straight with feet 6 inches apart. Hands open, arms at your sides. For extra safety stand in front of a chair.

Action

Shift your weight to your left leg as you lift your right toes and step forward on heel, then toes down.

Balance and step back.

Shift your right leg as you lift your left toes and step forward as before.

Balance and step back.

Do 10 times, alternating legs.

Verbal Cues

"Ready for ten."

"One… shift to left, right toes up and step forward… step back."

"Two… Shift to right, left toes up and step forward… then back."

"Three… Left, step, your arms relaxed… then back."

"Four… Right, step, feel your weight shift, good… then back."

"Five… Keep counting and shifting, toes up, step forward and rest."

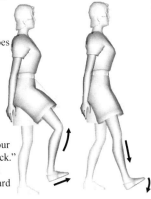

TABLE 10.3 — Exercises to Relieve Rigidity and Bradykinesia

- **Exercise to arise from chair**: Slide forward on the seat, leaning from the hips so that the body is at a 45° angle. Position one foot under the edge of the chair seat and the other foot one-half step forward. Next, position hands at the side of the seat near the front legs of the chair, and push with the arms while stepping forward, all in one continuous motion.

- **Exercise to sit down in a chair**: Reverse the process described for rising from the chair. Turn one's back to the chair, place one foot behind the other, bend the torso at a 45° angle, then sit slowly but smoothly while grasping the sides of the chair with the hands.

- **Exercise for stooped posture**: Stand with one's back to the wall, with the head, shoulders, buttocks, and heels all touching the wall. After holding the position for 30 seconds, walk away from the wall and then return, assuming the same position.

These exercises should be repeated 5 to 10 times every morning and evening to improve functional ability.

Goetz CG, et al. *Continuum*. 1995;1:121.

such as touching typewriter keys, before beginning more complex maneuvers. Patients may be taught to exaggerate movements by using a gross effort that extends too far and then, through practice, is refined into a smoother move. In this way, they can learn to handle faucets, doorknobs, and dressing and grooming activities. Lines painted on the floor can help patients step more regularly and may help to overcome freezing.

Symptoms of slowness and stiffness may be improved by repetitive movement exercises. First, the involved joint is moved passively; later, it is moved actively with assistance until eventually, it can be controlled by the patient.

223

■ **Gait Disturbance**

This problem is related to primary motoric disturbances as well as impairment of the ability to perform asymmetrical muscle contraction of the trunk. Patients have difficulty shifting weight from side to side. A focused approach to gait disorders involves particular attention to weight shifting, using exaggerated movements, to be practiced at home after initial instruction.

Hesitation when starting to walk (start hesitation) and the temporary inability to move (freezing) can sometimes be overcome by issuing verbal commands ("ready, set, go") to initiate movement and by learning to begin walking in a vigorous, sometimes marching fashion.

Patients with postural instability may begin walking with a few involuntary steps backward. Since these patients have a tendency to fall, their shoes should have leather, not rubber, soles and heel lifts to help tilt them forward.

Speech Therapy

A major source of disability in PD is disordered speech: hypophonia, dysarthria, and reduced variability in pitch and rhythm. Poor respiratory control also causes mumbled speech. Rigidity and bradykinesia involving the speech musculature aggravate all of these problems.

Other dyskinesias that may impair communication include:

- Tongue protrusion
- Lip smacking
- Grimacing
- Laryngeal stridor.

Although common late in the disease, speech and communication problems may appear early, particularly if the patient must speak at work. Thus early speech therapy may be helpful.

Speech therapy emphasizes breathing control; patients practice augmentation of voice loudness and variation in pitch. Exercises are intended to increase the number of words spoken with each breath. Patients may also find that reading or singing aloud is a good practice exercise. Watching lip and tongue movements in a mirror while speaking may help identify problems. A metronome may help patients to achieve measured speech.

Referral information regarding speech therapy for PD patients is available from the American Speech-Language-Hearing Association, 10801 Rockville Pike, Rockville, MD 20852. Phone: (301) 897-5700.

Occupational Therapy

Occupational therapy may emphasize general activities of daily living or specific adaptations intended to keep the patient working. Employment may be either the patient's usual premorbid occupation or a new type of work more appropriate for an individual with a movement disorder. Therapy usually includes exercises and other training to enhance fine motor coordination.

Many PD patients are able to remain employed for a long time, often through making selective adaptations or job changes.

Psychotherapy

The psychological changes that affect PD patients can be more devastating than the motor impairment, particularly early in the disease. Moreover, emotional stress can increase motor symptoms. Physicians, as well as family and friends, should consider the context in which the disease usually occurs. At a time when most people are looking forward to retirement, financial independence, and increased enjoyment of life, the newly diagnosed Parkinson patient faces the prospect of progressive disability, physical dependence, and high medical costs.

Not surprisingly, the most common psychological problem faced by these patients is depression. Primary-care physicians caring for PD patients often find it helpful to all concerned to refer patients and their families to a psychological counselor experienced with the mental and emotional problems of the disease. Selected reading materials for patients and families are shown in **Table 10**.**4**.

TABLE 10.4 — Selected Reading Materials for Parkinson's Disease Patients and Families

Parkinson's Disease: A Complete Guide for Patients and Families (Johns Hopkins Press Health Book). William J. Weiner, MD; 2001

300 Tips for Making Life with Parkinson's Disease Easier. Shelley Peterman Schwarz; 2002.

Answers to Frequently Asked Questions in Parkinson's Disease: A Resource Book for Patients and Families. David L Cram, MD; 2002.

Living Well, Running Hard: Lessons Learned from Living with Parkinson's Disease. John Ball; 2005

Parkinson's Disease and the Family: A New Guide (The Harvard University Press Family Health Guides). Nutan Sharma, MD, Elaine Richman, PhD; 2005.

The Parkinson's Disease Treatment Book: Partnering with Your Doctor to Get the Most from Your Medications. J Eric Ahlskog, MD; 2005.

Parkinson's Disease and the Art of Moving. John Argue. 2000.

A Life Shaken: My Encounter With Parkinson's Disease. Stephen Reich, MD; 2004.

Preventive measures are particularly important for patients diagnosed with PD because later diagnosis and treatment of dental disease becomes increasingly difficult.[3] A number of medications, including anticholinergics and antidepressants, commonly prescribed for Parkinson's patients cause xerostomia (dry mouth) by suppressing the production of saliva, thus reducing its antibacterial and cleansing actions, resulting in an increased risk for coronal and root surface caries, periodontal disease, and tongue erosion. Chemically induced xerostomia is sometimes employed to reduce drooling in patients with sialorrhea.

Saliva is also important because it dissolves food particles, thus allowing keener taste sensations, aiding digestion, and lubricating the food bolus for easier swallowing. It also lubricates oral tissues and facilitates clear speech.

The "on-off" phenomena, when associated with dyskinetic movements, twisting of trunk or limbs, and writhing of the tongue and lips, can pose problems for both patient and dentist. However, improved techniques and new restorative and prosthetic materials make it possible to perform procedures that were not feasible for these patients 2 decades ago.

Denture retention depends to a large extent on appropriate muscle function. Tremors or dyskinesias affecting the tongue may dislodge a mandibular denture, and rigid and uncontrolled facial muscles may prevent the maxillary denture from maintaining a good retentive seal. Furthermore, elderly patients or those who have been edentulous for many years lack a bony ridge height for dentures to rest on, affecting the ability to keep them in place.

The use of local anesthesia is not contraindicated in patients with PD, although demerol probably should not be prescribed for patients taking selegiline since a rare interaction has been reported. Concomitant medical problems, such as heart disease and hypertension, should be considered by dentists in planning treatment and anesthesia.

Levodopa was once thought to cause softening of tooth enamel and, in turn, an increased incidence of caries. The increased tendency to tooth decay in Parkinson's patients is now thought to be the result of xerostomia and the decreased ability to perform regular oral hygiene.

New varieties of electric and sonic toothbrushes facilitate dental care for Parkinson patients. Flossing between teeth is made easier by floss holders. Optimum results require brushing the teeth with a fluoride and tartar-control dentifrice after meals and before retiring at night. Dilute fluoride rinses, such as neutral sodium fluoride solution or a stannous fluoride tablet dissolved in water, are sold without prescription and can be used daily as a 1-minute rinse to protect the teeth. (The solution should not be swallowed.) In choosing a mouthwash, patients should avoid those that contain alcohol, which increases drying of the oral mucous membrane.

Family Counseling

Parkinson's disease has implications for virtually all facets of the family's life and future security.[2] Common family reactions include anger and concomitant guilt, depression, fatigue, and social isolation. Helping the family or caregivers to understand PD and what it must mean to the patient can be helpful. Some physicians keep a lending library of books on the disease for this purpose.

Family members or caregivers should be encouraged to accompany patients on physician visits. Support groups for patients and their families, which are widely available, provide patients with opportunities to share information about the disease and available services, about new books, therapies, and aids to daily living. Such groups also offer psychological support and sounding boards about the more troublesome aspects of the disease.

Physicians should help ensure that patients and their families are using all available community resources. Valuable sources of information include the leading national foundations devoted to PD, which provide newsletters, books, and general information regarding the disease (**Table 10.2**). Foundations can also guide patients and families to resources within their own communities.

Nonpharmacologic Approach to Associated Disorders

■ Swallowing Problems and Sialorrhea

These disorders may develop at any stage of PD and can be thoroughly evaluated by a speech therapist. Symptoms may include:

- Choking
- Coughing
- Drooling
- Holding food in the mouth.

Motor problems contributing to these difficulties include:

- Decreased tongue mobility
- Decreased elevation of the larynx
- Impaired swallowing reflex
- Diminished pharyngeal peristalsis.

Patients may fail to swallow saliva automatically, resulting in pooling in the mouth and throat. Saliva buildup may also contribute to muffled speech.

Careful attention to the process of swallowing may help improve sialorrhea and related problems. Patients should be advised to consciously swallow saliva frequently. Holding the head upright helps to prevent pooling and enhances the swallowing mechanism. Finally, a conscious effort to swallow saliva must be made before speaking.

Patients should also think through each step of chewing and swallowing. They should eat slowly, taking only small amounts of food with each bite. Food should be chewed thoroughly and swallowed before the next bite is taken. Some patients may require video fluoroscopic evaluation of swallowing and, possibly, may need placement of a percutaneous esophagogastrostomy tube.

There have been recent reports of botulinum toxin injections into the parotid glands improving excess saliva. However, this procedure is not approved by most insurance companies.

■ Nutritional Disturbances

Patients often have trouble preparing food, and eating or swallowing. In frustration, they may consume a very restricted diet, a problem enhanced by coexisting depression or dementia. Dietary consultation is often useful. However, certain general considerations can be emphasized by physicians, including:

- The diet should include all food groups.
- Caloric intake should be sufficient to maintain body weight.
- Include sufficient fiber and fluid to prevent constipation and enough calcium to avoid osteoporosis.

Specific dietary considerations for PD patients include:

- Patients with motor fluctuations may find that the medication is more effective if taken 30 minutes before meals. This is due to protein competition for transport with levodopa.

- Patients with severe fluctuations may eliminate protein during the day to avoid this competition. All protein needs are then provided at dinner.

■ Constipation

Both the inactivity inherent in PD and the drugs taken to control its manifestations can lead to constipation (see Chapter 9, *Complications of Parkinson's Disease and Its Therapy*). Gastrointestinal autonomic dysfunction may contribute as well. Management includes:

- Regular physical exercise
- Adequate intake of water and dietary fiber
- Use of stool softeners.

■ Seborrheic Dermatitis

Although the cause of seborrheic dermatitis and the reasons for its association with PD are unknown, effective therapies to provide symptomatic relief and control are available. Characterized by excessive sebum production by sebaceous glands and rapid skin cell turnover, seborrheic dermatitis leads to an inflammatory response that manifests as patchy or scaly, reddened, itchy skin. On the scalp, the condition may be simple dandruff or can involve the whole spectrum of signs and symptoms.

Although patients with PD tend to have long-term problems with seborrheic dermatitis, levodopa tends to resolve the condition or decrease its severity. The explanation seems to be that levodopa decreases sebaceous gland activity.

The condition can usually be treated with over-the-counter medications, including:

- Neutral or bland acne soap
- Ketoconazole shampoo
- Shampoos and lotions containing selenium (used as directed, two or three times a week, since they may cause hair loss with excessive use)
- Shampoos, lotions, and creams containing pyrithione zinc.

■ Sexuality

There is little written on the impact of PD on sexual function. There have been some reports in both male and female populations showing that there exists more dysfunction in the PD population compared with controls.[4] In males, erectile dysfunction is most commonly described. **Table 10.5** lists the impact of PD on sexual functioning.[5] In a study devoted exclusively to women,[6] it was found that women have anxiety, inhibition, and other concerns as noted in **Table 10.6**.

In most studies involving men, the problems listed in **Table 10.7** are described. In a recent open-label study, ten men had improved sexual function with the use of sildenafil (Viagra), 50 mg per encounter.[6] No significant side effects were reported after eight encounters.

Levodopa may induce feelings of well-being, and in some patients, results in a significant but generally short-lived increase in sexuality. Hypersexuality has also been described with dopaminergic therapy. Due to the great embarrassment caused by these behaviors, it may be difficult for family members to report them. It is the responsibility of the physician to initiate this discussion.[4] Treatment of hypersexuality includes counseling, lowering of the dose of medication, and the possible use of an atypical antipsychotic agent.

TABLE 10.5 — Impact of Parkinson's Disease on Sexual Functioning

- Caregiver strain
- Physical unattractiveness
- Abnormal movements
- Excessive sweating
- Excessive salivation
- Motor features
- Depression in patient
- Impotence

Lambert D, et al. *Clin Neurosci.* 1998;5:73-77.

TABLE 10.6 — Problems Reported by Women With Parkinson's Disease

- Anxiety* ($P = 0.04$)
- Inhibition* ($P = 0.04$)
- Vaginal tightness* ($P = 0.03$)
- Involuntary urination* ($P = 0.03$)
- Health problems interfere with sex
- Dissatisfaction with body appearance

* Statistically significant.

Lambert D, et al. *Clin Neurosci.* 1998;5:75.

TABLE 10.7 — Common Features of Male Sexual Dysfunction

- Noncommunication
- Dissatisfaction
- Premature ejaculation
- Impotence
- Infrequency of sexual act

Lambert D, et al. *Clin Neurosci.* 1998;5:75.

REFERENCES

1. Golbe LI, Sage JI. Medical treatment of Parkinson's disease. In: Kurlan R, ed. *Treatment of Movement Disorders*. Philadelphia, Pa: JB Lippincott Co; 1995:1-56.

2. Goetz CG, Jankovic J, Koller WC, et al. Nonpharmacological approaches to the management of Parkinson's disease. *Continuum*. 1995;1:114-129.

3. Paulson RB, Paulson GW. Dental considerations for the Parkinson's patient. *Parkinson Report*. 1997;19:23-26.

4. Lambert D, Waters CH. Sexual dysfunction in Parkinson's disease. *Clin Neurosci*. 1998;5:73-77.

5. Welsh M, Hung L, Waters CH. Sexuality in women with Parkinson's disease. *Mov Disord*. 1997;12:923-927.

6. Zesiewicz TA, Helal M, Hauser RA. Sildenafil citrate (Viagra) for the treatment of erectile dysfunction in men with Parkinson's disease. *Mov Disord*. 2000;15:305-308.

11   Surgery

Surgical procedures for Parkinson's disease (PD) declined rapidly with the introduction of levodopa. Recently, however, interest in surgery has been rekindled as a result of problems with chronic levodopa treatment of this relentlessly progressive disease. Tremor is variably responsive to medication. Many patients develop drug-associated motor fluctuations and dyskinesias, and symptoms that are not amenable to medication, such as postural instability and freezing, emerge over time.

In addition to and perhaps because of these shortcomings of medical intervention, there have been major advances in stereotactic surgery, including:

- Improved instrumentation with more precise target localization
- Computed tomography (CT)- and magnetic resonance imaging (MRI)-guided localization
- Intraoperative electrophysiologic monitoring and stimulation techniques that permit reversible disruption of neuronal function
- New awareness of functional anatomy, resulting in identification of more rational targets
- Advances in transplant biology that suggest the possibility of implanting dopamine-producing cells.

Surgical procedures for PD can be conceptually divided into those aimed at reducing abnormal neuronal activity and those seeking to augment and restore dopaminergic tone (**Table 11.1**).[1] Targets for the ablative and stimulation procedures include the thalamus, the globus pallidus internus (GPi) and the subthalamic

TABLE 11.1 — Surgical Procedures for Parkinson's Disease

Reduction of Abnormal Neuronal Activity	Augmentation of Dopaminergic Tone

• Thermo-lesion
• Deep brain stimulation
• Gamma knife radiation
	• Tissue grafts:
	  – Fetal mesencephalic
	  – Other tissue:
	    › Carotid body cells
	    › Sympathetic ganglion cells
	    › Pigmented retinal cells
	• Nerve growth factor infusion
	• Gene therapy

Target	**Target**
• Thalamus (Vim/Vop) • Globus Pallidus internus (GPi) • Subthalamic nucleus (STN)	• Striatum • Substantia nigra (SN)

Abbreviations: Vim, video-intensification microscopy; Vop, venous occlusion plethysmography.

Adapted from: Metman LV, O'Leary ST. *Mov Disord.* 2005;20(suppl 11):S45-S56.

nucleus (STN). Targets for the restorative procedures involve the striatum and substantia nigra (SN).

A wide variety of neurosurgical operations have been proposed over the years for the treatment of PD, many of which are now obsolete. Currently, the most popular techniques are:

- Thalamotomy
- Pallidotomy
- Chronic deep-brain stimulation (DBS) of the ventral intermediate (Vim) nucleus of the thalamus, STN, and GPi, using an implantable pulse generator (IPG).

In addition to these ablative and stimulation approaches to treatment of PD, in the past decade, there have been advances in the development of neurorestorative procedures, including fetal and stem cell transplantation, gene therapy, and infusion of various neural growth factors. Current information on the efficacy and safety of the currently used and evolving procedures are discussed below.

Ablative Procedures

The basic technique of pallidal and thalamic surgery is similar.[2] Whether a lesion is to be made or DBS performed, the procedure is identical down to the point at which either a lesion is made or the stimulator is implanted. The procedures are done using MRI guidance with the patient in the "off" state, under local anesthesia, and the Elekta Leksell G frame in place. The stereotactic three-dimensional coordinates of the anterior and posterior commissures are determined using the scanner's computer software. The desired target is chosen, its stereotactic coordinates are read off, and the patient is taken to the operating room.

The bulk of the operating time is taken up in physiologic confirmation of the target site, using a microelectrode advanced to the selected target. Continuous recording or microstimulation every 1 mm is carried out along the trajectory, starting 10 mm to 15 mm above and extending a variable distance into or through the target.[2] Up to four trajectories, 2 mm to 3 mm apart, and six trajectories, 2 mm apart, are usually sufficient in pallidal and thalamic exploration, respectively.

When a neuron is encountered, it is studied for any receptive field (RF) by applying tactile (hair-bending, light touch, deep pressure) or thermal stimuli, passive joint bending, muscle compression, auditory, or visual stimuli, and by asking the patient to carry out voluntary movements on the contralateral side of the body. In the case of pallidal units, there may also be ipsilateral movement-related RFs. The locations of RFs are mapped out on body diagrams called figurine charts, visual responses on maps of the visual fields. Projected fields (PFs) are similarly mapped by determining the effects of threshold stimulation (up to 100 mA). The electrode's position may be confirmed with an image intensifier showing the tip at the location of the central beam in a sagittal view.

Deep-brain stimulation electrodes are attached to a temporary transcutaneous cable for short-term stimulation before internalization to insert a radio frequency-coupled, battery-powered, totally programmable IPG.

Pallidotomy

Modern pallidotomy is based on a prospective strategy aimed at restoring functional alterations in neuronal circuitry consequent to degeneration of dopamine neurons in the substantia nigra pars compacta (SNc) (**Figure 11.1**).[3]

In the 1950s, pallidotomy with a target site in the anterodorsal part of the pallidum became a popular procedure for PD. Thalamotomy soon replaced

FIGURE 11.1 — Basal Ganglia Circuitry

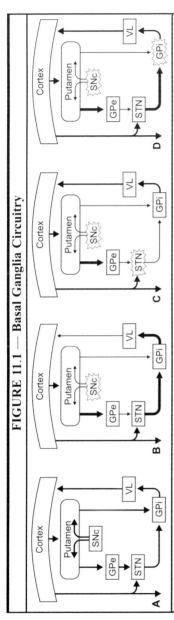

In normal basal ganglia circuitry, output from the gobus pallidus interna (GPi) exerts a chronic inhibitory effect on thalamocortical and brain stem neurons. Activation of the direct pathways inhibits firing of the GPi, whereas activation of the indirect pathway stimulates it. Dopamine from the substantia nigra pars compacta (SNc) stimulates the direct and inhibits the indirect pathway *(A)*. In Parkinson's disease, loss of striatal dopamine secondary to degeneration of SNc neurons dimishes inhibition of the GPi by the direct pathway and increases excitation of the GPi by the indirect connection. Increased GPi output results, in turn, in inhibition of thalamo-cortical and brain stem neurons *(B)*. A lesion of the subthalamic nucleus (STN) diminishes the excessive excitatory stimulation of the GPi, consequently reducing the inhibitory outflow to brain stem and thalamocortical pathways *(C)*. A lesion of the GPi directly diminishes its inhibitory output *(D)*.

Adapted from: Kurlan R, ed. *Treatment of Movement Disorders*. Philadelphia, Pa: JB Lippincott Co; 1995:57-93.

11

pallidotomy as procedure of choice, however, because it was believed to relieve tremor more consistently and to be associated with a lower rate of symptom recurrence. Tremor and rigidity were reported to recur in 25% of patients after pallidal surgery compared with only 11% after thalamotomy.

In 1992, posteroventral pallidotomy in 38 patients whose main complaint was hypokinesia was reported to produce long-lasting tremor relief, complete or almost complete relief of rigidity and hypokinesia, and improvement in speech, gait, dystonia, and levodopa-induced dyskinesias.[4,5] But adverse effects included central homonymous visual-field defects in 14% of patients and one instance of transitory facial weakness and dysphasia, reflections of damage to the optic tract and internal capsule, which lie in close proximity to the GPi.

Now well studied, pallidotomy is associated with great reduction in dyskinesias (>80%) and a 30% improvement in motor scores. The major results are contralateral. The improvement, if any, in gait and balance is short-lived.

Thirty-seven patients were assigned to either unilateral pallidotomy or to best medical treatment followed by pallidotomy 6 months later.[6] At the 6 month-time point, UPDRS-III "off" scores improved by 31% in the pallidotomy group, and worsened by 8% in the medical control group. Pallidotomy also improved dyskinesias and diaries showed that "on-time without dyskinesias" improved by 2.8 hrs versus 0.3 hrs in the medical control group.

Long-term follow-up of unilateral pallidotomy in advanced PD has recently been reported. In a follow up study of 20 of the 40 patients who underwent unilateral surgery and were available for analysis, overall function continued to be better than baseline. Tremor, bradykinesia, and "on" dyskinesia sustained improvement.[7]

240

The short- and long-term benefit of unilateral pallidotomy were assessed in a more recent single-blind trial that randomized patients to receive unilateral pallidotomy (n = 18) or best medical therapy (n = 18).[8] At the 6-month follow up, patients who received surgery exhibited a significant reduction (32% decrease) in the total UPDRS score compared with medical treatment (5% increase). Surgical patients also showed improvement in all of the cardinal signs of PD including tremor, rigidity, bradykinesia, gait, and balance. Drug-induced dyskinesias were also markedly improved. Twenty patients were followed for 2 years to assess the effect of time on clinical outcome. Improvements in the total UPDRS scores, *off* motor, and complications of therapy subscores were sustained in these patients.

The most recent multicenter, single-blind, randomized trial compared unilateral pallidotomy with bilateral STN DBS in 34 patients with advanced PD.[9] Of the 14 patients randomized to the unilateral pallidotomy group, 13 completed the 6-month follow-up. Their UPDRS-III "off" scores improved by 20% compared with baseline and the severity but not duration of dyskinesias improved. In the head-to-head comparison, unilateral pallidotomy was found to be less effective than bilateral STN DBS in reducing parkinsonian symptoms (UPDRS-III) and reducing the dyskinesia duration. Both treatments improved dyskinesia severity.

According to the most recent Evidence-Based Medical (EBM) review of surgical treatments of PD, unilateral pallidotomy was classified as *efficacious* and *clinically useful* as a symptomatic adjunct to levodopa and *likely efficacious* and *clinically useful* in the treatment of motor complications.[10]

■ Patient Selection

Candidates for pallidotomy are patients with medically intractable PD as defined by significant motor morbidity not optimally managed by medication. Features responsive to pallidotomy are:

- Motor fluctuations
- "On-off" phenomena
- Dystonia ("off" or "on")
- Drug-induced dyskinesia.

Additional criteria include:[11]

- Demonstration of a clear and long-lasting benefit from antiparkinson medication, levodopa and dopamine agonists in particular
- Treatment of any existing depression
- Thorough assessment of patients' cognitive state. (Those with significant cognitive decline may be unable to cooperate with motor and visual field testing during the procedure and are less likely to have long-lasting improvement.)

Thalamotomy

Stereotactic thalamotomy was introduced in the 1950s, with lesions created by chemicals, heat, or freezing.[3] The procedure became a regular treatment for prominent unilateral tremor in PD. Follow-up studies were usually short-term and the majority were unblinded. However, in one blinded study, an evaluation of 17 patients in long-term follow-up (mean, 10.9 years after unilateral or subthalamotomy), investigators used videotapes and the UPDRS to compare tremor ipsilateral and contralateral to the side of surgery.[12] (A sign of long-term efficacy would be reversal of tremor side dominance.)

Tremor was found to be significantly less in the upper extremity contralateral to the operated side, indicating that stereotactic thalamotomy improved the absolute magnitude or ameliorated the rate of progression of tremor.

It seems clear that the procedure can improve contralateral tremor (45% to 92% of patients) and, to a lesser extent, rigidity (41% to 92%).[3] Bilateral thalamotomies are reported to improve tremor in 33% to 73% of patients and rigidity in 22% to 74%. Thalamotomy generally does not improve bradykinesia, akinesia, postural instability, and ipsilateral tremor.[11]

Complications of thalamotomy have included:

- Contralateral hemiparesis (0.5% to 26% of patients) can be minimized with modern stereotactic techniques and use of microelectrode recording
- Seizures (<1.3%)
- Paresthesias, usually of lips or fingers (1% to 3%)
- Uncommonly, ataxia, apraxia, hypotonia, abulia, gait disturbances
- Perioperative mortality (0.4% to 6%) usually due to hemorrhage at lesion site. Mortality in the modern era is expected to be <1%.

Bilateral thalamotomy is associated with a higher incidence of complications, including:

- Speech and swallowing problems, particularly in those with preoperative dysfunction
- Worsening of dysarthria in 29% of patients.

Modern stereotactic techniques and staged procedures have improved but not eliminated these complications. Therefore, given the high rate of cognitive and speech problems associated with bilateral thalamotomies, and the success and lower incidence of complications of pallidotomy and DBS, thalamotomy is generally not recommended as a first choice procedure.[11]

■ **Patient Selection**

In tremor-predominant patients, several points need to be considered. Given the progressive nature of PD, patients' potential for developing other functionally disabling symptoms must be weighed against the likelihood and relative degree of improvement in tremor after thalamotomy versus other procedures aimed at the pallidum or subthalamic nuclei.

Deep-Brain Stimulation

Chronic high-frequency thalamic stimulation has recently been described as an alternative to thalamotomy for the treatment of tremor in PD.[3] A stimulation frequency of 100 Hz to 250 Hz is generally employed, coupled with a pulse width of 60 to 210 microseconds. The current intensity or voltage necessary to alleviate tremor may increase progressively during the first months after surgery, presumably due to the development of fibrosis and increased resistance around the electrode tip, and must be adjusted accordingly. When stimulation is effective, tremor reduction occurs within 3 seconds, and the effect is lost within seconds of the stimulator being turned off. A rebound worsening lasting from a few minutes to several hours has been observed after discontinuation of chronic stimulation.

Previously used safely as a palliative for intractable pain related to somatosensory deafferentation and various movement disorders, chronic high-frequency thalamic stimulation was originally proposed as a less risky treatment than a second, contralateral procedure for patients with disabling tremor who had undergone a previous thalamotomy; if stimulation of the side opposite the original lesion caused complications, it could be turned off.

A multicenter study of high-frequency, unilateral thalamic stimulation involved 29 patients with essential tremor and 24 with PD, 18 of whom had bilateral tremor.[13]

Stimulation was initiated 1 day postoperatively unless the patient exhibited a microthalamotomy effect (defined as tremor reduction with the IPG off, assumed to be due to the trauma of electrode placement). Patients were instructed on how to switch the device on and off with a hand-held magnet and to turn it off at night to preserve the battery and reduce the possibility of tolerance. Medication for PD (levodopa, 23 patients; dopamine agonists, 17; anticholinergics, 5) was held constant for at least 1 month before enrollment and during the first 3 months of the study.

Follow-up included a blinded evaluation 3 months postsurgery with patients randomized to stimulation "on" or "off" and 6-, 9-, and 12-month open-label follow-up assessments. Evaluations consisted of:

- The UPDRS motor examination
- Global assessment of disability by both patient and examiner on a scale from 0 to 4
- Writing a sentence, drawing a spiral (see Chapter 4, *Etiology*), drawing a straight line between lines, pouring liquid
- Patients' subjective assessment of change from baseline to 3 months (marked, moderate, mild improvement, worsening, no change).

At the 3-month blinded evaluation and at 6-, 9-, and 12-month open-label assessments, results were:

- A significant decrease contralaterally in the clinical rating of tremor in stimulation "on" (**Figure 11.2**)
- Total resolution of their target tremors in 14 (58.3%) PD patients and 9 (31%) of those with essential tremor; one (4.2%) PD patient and one (3.4%) essential tremor patient had no change
- No effect observed in limb ipsilateral to the IPG
- Efficacy was not reduced at 1 year.

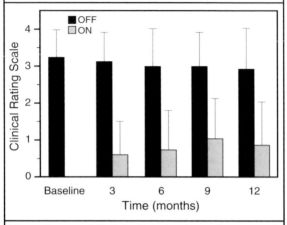

FIGURE 11.2 — Change in Parkinsonian Tremor With Chronic Thalamic Stimulation

Shown here are blinded, clinical ratings of tremor at 3 months and open-label evaluations at 6, 9, and 12 months in Parkinson's disease patients with implantable pulse generators (IPGs) switched to "on."

Koller W, et al. *Ann Neurol.* 1997;42:292-299.

Complications related to surgery were few. Stimulation was associated with transient paresthesias lasting several seconds, which occurred in most patients at 3 months. Complications related to the device that occurred during the first year were:

- Incisional skin infection (two patients) successfully treated with antibiotics
- IPG malfunction necessitating replacement (one patient)
- Extension wire erosion necessitating replacement (one patient).

Beneficial effects have been noted through 5-year follow-ups of the early trials.[3] Although not studied in a systematic way, chronic stimulation may also improve rigidity, unilateral pain, and dyskinesia. Akinesia appears to be unchanged. Adverse effects (paresthesias, dystonia, gait disorders, dysarthria) have been mild and generally resolve when stimulation is discontinued. In a recent report, thalamic stimulation resulted in contralateral improvement of parkinsonian rigidity and slowness.[14]

The principal advantage of thalamic stimulation is its potential to provide functional benefit without the creation of an irreversible lesion, particularly important in patients who:

- Are older
- Have bilateral tremor
- Have undergone an earlier contralateral thalamotomy
- Have a preexisting speech disorder.

The procedure's principal disadvantages include:

- The possibility that the system will need replacement because of fracture or infection
- Battery requires replacement after several years. (May be obviated by development of externally rechargeable stimulators).
- Progression of other features of PD are not improved by this procedure.

Although the mechanism of action of electrical stimulation of the Vim is not known, it may:

- Create functional ablation of a "firing center" or
- Serve to desynchronize abnormal depolarizations that have become overactive and autonomous.

Deep-brain stimulators have more recently been implanted in the GPi and STN to treat other motor signs of PD.[15] Both have been reported to improve all of the cardinal motor symptoms, including tremor. However, stimulation in the STN has also been reported to induce dyskinesias at higher current intensities.

The effects of GPi stimulation on parkinsonian motor signs may be mediated by mechanisms similar to those proposed for thalamic stimulation. Assuming the improvement is a result of decreased GPi output, it can result either through inhibition or blocking of neuronal activity:

- Directly via depolarization block; or
- Indirectly via antidromic activation of globus pallidus externa (GPe).

Similarly, STN stimulation has a host of possible mechanisms that underlie its beneficial effects on parkinsonian motor signs, including:

- Direct inactivation
- Indirect inactivation by alteration of GPi neuronal activity (decreasing it, blocking its transmission, or normalizing its pattern)
- Antidromic activation of GPe leading to inhibition of STN, GPi, and/or reticularis neurons in thalamus, leading, in turn, to normalization of thalamic neuronal activity.

Bilateral STN stimulation was performed in 24 patients with idiopathic PD.[16] One-year evaluation revealed 60% improvement in "off" scores. The mean dose of dopaminergic medication was reduced by half. One complication included an intracerebral hematoma resulting in paralysis and aphasia.

Twenty-four patients with advanced PD underwent bilateral STN stimulation.[17] These patients averaged 55 years of age with 16.3 years of PD and they were taking 1265-mg equivalents of levodopa. They suffered from a variety of dyskinesias. This study focused on the potential reduction of dyskinesia. There was good benefit from the surgery with respect to many features of PD as seen in **Figure 11.3**. Sixty percent of patients no

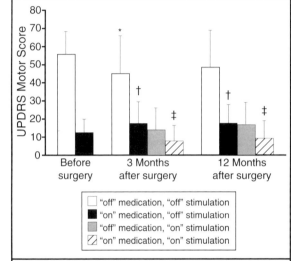

FIGURE 11.3 — Motor Examination Before and After Bilateral Subthalamic Nucleus Stimulation for Parkinson's Disease

Legend:
- "off" medication, "off" stimulation
- "on" medication, "off" stimulation
- "off" medication, "on" stimulation
- "on" medication, "on" stimulation

Mean ± SD motor examination score (Unified Parkinson's Disease Rating Scale [UPDRS] Part III) in the "off" medication and "on" medication conditions before and 3 and 12 months after surgery. After surgery, the UPDRS motor score was also evaluated in the "off" stimulation and "on" stimulation conditions.

* $P <0.004$ For the comparison with the "off" medication condition before surgery.

† $P <0.001$ for the comparison with the "off" stimulation and "off" medication condition.

‡ $P <0.001$ for the comparison with the "off" stimulation and "On" medication condition.

Fraix V, et al. *Neurology.* 2000;55:1923.

longer had dyskinesia. The "off" period dystonia score also improved. The levodopa dose was significantly reduced from 952 ± 509 mg to 184 ± 190 mg at 12 months. The improvement in motor condition allowed for this dramatic reduction in levodopa requirements.

A small randomized, single-blind, 12-month study compared DBS in the STN or in the GPi in 10 PD patients with levodopa-induced dyskinesias and response fluctuations.[18] Patients and evaluating clinicians were blinded as to stimulation site. When off levodopa, both GPi and STN groups showed a similar response, with approximately 40% improvement in UPDRS scores. Rigidity, tremor, and bradykinesia improved in both groups. In combination with levodopa, there was greater improvement in the GPi group. DBS at either site reduced levodopa-induced dyskinesias, although medication requirement was reduced only in the STN group.

In a subsequent trial, DBS was performed bilaterally in the STN in 96 patients and GPi in 38 patients in a multicenter study. At 3 months, a blinded crossover evaluation was performed. The investigators and patients were unaware of the status of stimulation (on or off) or sequence of evaluation. Both locations proved to be very efficacious. Improvement was shown in motor function without dyskinesias. Adverse events include seven intracranial hemorrhages and one infection.[19]

A 2-day random-ordered protocol was used to evaluate the efficacy of DBS in the STN after 6 to 8 months (n = 14).[20] Stimulation was activated and deactivated in a randomized double-blind crossover fashion. Unfortunately the study cohort was not homogeneous. Bilateral DBS was performed in nine patients and unilateral in five patients who had predominately unilateral symptoms. In addition, three of the patients had previous procedures. The data were only reported for the 14 patients as a group. However, at the 6 to 8 month time point, the improvement in the UPDRS-III was 27%. The effect on motor complications was more striking. Dyskinesia measured with the UPDRS-IV improved by 41% and motor fluctuations by 33% as documented with patient/caregiver diaries.

Østergaard and colleagues used a similar randomized, double-blind crossover design in a recent study of 26 PD patients who underwent bilateral STN stimulation.[21] After 12 months, bilateral STN DBS improved UPDRS-III "off" scores by 64%, dyskinesia duration was reduced by 86%, and percent of the waking day spent in "off" state improved by 83%.

As discussed previously, a recent study compared the effect of unilateral pallidotomy with that of bilateral STN stimulation in a randomized, single-blind trial.[9] After 6 months, and at 12 hours after medications were withheld, the UPDRS motor assessment was improved in both groups with a significantly greater improvement with bilateral STN stimulation (median improvement, 25 vs 9.5 points; $P = 0.002$). These changes represent a relative improvement over baseline of 49% versus 20% with unilateral pallidotomy. Duration but not severity of dyskinesias was improved to a larger extent with STN DBS than with unilateral pallidotomy.

The principal advantages and disadvantages of DBS are listed in **Table 11.2**.[22]

Surgical and hardware-related complications associated STN DBS procedures were recently reported by Lyons and colleagues.[23] A chart review was conducted on PD 80 patients (average disease duration 12.5 years from diagnosis) who underwent 160 unilateral or bilateral procedures from 1997 to 2002. There were no deaths or persistent neurologic sequelae in any PF the patients in this series. Surgical complications included:

- Procedure aborted (4.9% of patients; 2.5% of procedures)

TABLE 11.2 — Advantages and Disadvantages of Deep Brain Stimulation

Advantages
- Immediate symptomatic and functional improvement
- Stimulation is adjustable and can be "customized"
- Lower risk of lesion-related complications
- Lower risk with bilateral procedure

Disadvantages
- Long-term outcome unclear
- Replacement of batteries
- Implantation of a foreign body (hardware)
- Cost to the patient and the neurologist
- Limited coverage by Medicare and other insurance carriers

Adapted from: Jankovic J. 11th Annual Course. A Comprehensive Review of Movement Disorders for the Clinical Practitioner. Aspen, Colo; August 3-6, 2001.

- Intraoperative intracranial bleed (1.2% of patients; 0.6% of procedures)
- Seizures (1.2% of patients; 0.6% of procedures)
- Infection requiring removal of complete DBS system (2.5% of patients; 1.9% of procedures)
- Infections requiring removal of the IPG (3.7% of patients; 1.9% of procedures)
- Misplaced leads (12.5% of patients; 9.0% of procedures).

Hardware-related complications included:
- Lead replacements due to fracture or migration (8.8% of patients; 4.5% of procedures)
- Extension-wire replacements (3.8% of patients; 1.9% of procedures)
- Implantable pulse generator complications (20% of patients; 12.9% of procedures), approximately 75% of which were due to malfunction.

Transplantation Procedures

■ Fetal Nigral Transplantation

From a scientific perspective, fetal nigral grafts have been the most consistent and best donor cells for transplantation.

Transplant Material

Fetal mesencephalic cells can be transplanted as either a cell suspension, used in most studies to date, or as solid grafts.[24] Cell-suspension grafts provide more homogeneous tissue distribution but necessitate pooling of tissue, and infection or rejection in any one donor could adversely affect all graft deposits. Solid grafts, on the other hand, have an extended donor window, are easier to prepare, and preserve cytoarchitectural relationships. The preparations have shown comparable survival.

Implantation Site

Grafts may be implanted into the putamen, caudate, or both.[24] The postcommissural putamen is considered a good primary site for several reasons, including:

- Both autopsy and positron emission tomography (PET) scan studies demonstrate greater dopamine depletion within the posterior putamen than in the anterior putamen-caudate nucleus complex in Parkinson's patients.
- Degeneration of the SNc in PD preferentially occurs in regions that project to the posterior putamen.
- Experiments in methylphenyltetrahydropyridine (MPTP)-lesioned primates demonstrate that dopamine grafts placed exclusively into the putamen induce significant improvement of motor function.

The anterior putamen-caudate nucleus may also be an important target, however, because:

- Hemiparkinsonism can be induced by MPTP injection into the caudate nucleus.
- Fetal nigral grafts placed into the caudate nucleus of MPTP-treated monkeys can induce significant functional recovery, with benefits different from those associated with grafting into the posterior putamen.

The best clinical results may ultimately be associated with grafting into both caudate and putamen or into other potential target areas, such as the SNc and the nucleus accumbens.

Immunosuppression

Although immunosuppression is not essential in the immunologically privileged central nervous system, surgical trauma or the graft itself could disrupt the blood-brain barrier and permit the immune system access to graft antigens.[24] Thus most transplant groups treat study patients with cyclosporin A (CsA) for varying periods before and after the procedure. The absence of evidence of immune rejection 1 year after discontinuation of CsA has suggested that prolonged immunosuppression may not be necessary. In any case, the need for immunosuppression after fetal transplantation remains controversial.

Clinical Findings

In 13 patients (two with MPTP-induced parkinsonism), PET documented increased fluorodopa uptake in the grafted striatum compared with preoperative levels. This finding indicates that grafted dopamine neurons can survive and grow in the human parkinsonian brain. Moreover, autopsy findings in two patients who died from unrelated events 18 and 19 months, respectively, after transplantation strengthened this hypothesis by revealing robust survival of transplanted neurons, with reinnervation of the postcommissural putamen.[25]

Results have been inconsistent and difficult to compare, however, because of:

- Variations in patient selection
- Transplant variables
- Rating systems
- Level of scrutiny
- Clinical expertise.

The early success of human fetal cell transplantation reported in several unblinded case series prompted two large, blinded, controlled trials. Freed and coworkers randomly assigned 40 patients to undergo transplantation or sham surgery.[26] Patients who received sham surgery were offered formal transplants after 1 year. The outcomes were analyzed by dividing the groups into younger (<60 years of age) and older patients. The younger patients who received a transplant had a significant improvement in "off" UPDRS scores ($P = 0.010$) compared with those in the sham group. The older patients showed no benefit. The Schwab and England Activity Scale also showed improvement in this same group. The fluorodopa PET scans showed significant increases at 1 year in the transplanted group regardless of age. One patient had a subdural hematoma 2 months after surgery. Two patients died. Large numbers of dopamine fibers were seen in the transplant tracks. In both autopsies, fiber outgrowth was seen. Long-term follow-up of these patients revealed a troublesome occurrence. Five patients have developed disabling dyskinesias even with a reduction or elimination of parkinsonian drugs. These five patients were all in the younger group (<60 years).

More recently, Olanow et al reported the results of a 24-month, double-blind, controlled trial in 34 patients with advanced PD.[27] Patients were randomized to receive bilateral fetal nigral transplantation with one or four donors per side, or a placebo procedure. The primary end point was change between baseline and final visit in the motor component of the UPDRS. There was no significant treatment effect; patients in the placebo and one-donor groups deteriorated over the 24 months of follow up, whereas those in the four-donor group improved. Pairwise comparisons were not significant. Despite evidence of significant striatal fluorodopa uptake, 56% of transplanted patients developed dyskinesia that persisted after overnight withdrawal of dopaminergic medication ("off"-medication dyskinesia). No placebo treated patients developed this unusual type of dyskinesia (since termed "runaway dyskinesias") that, in some cases, was severely disabling and required another surgical intervention.

■ Pigmented Retinal Cells

Researchers have attempted to find alternatives to fetal mesencephalic cells as transplant tissue. Human retinal pigmented epithelial (hRPE) cells have been studied in this regard. To date, one open-label pilot study has been reported.[28] In this study, six patients received unilateral, stereotactic, putaminal placement of hRPE cells attached to biocompatible microcarriers. No immunosuppression was used. Six months postoperatively, there was a 34% improvement in the primary outcome measure, the UPDRS-III. Additionally, secondary outcome measures were improved, including the total-UPDRS and Schwab and England score. No "runaway" or levodopa-independent dyskinesias were identified and, in fact, half of the patients had lower dyskinesia scores postoperatively. Although these early results are promising, it should be noted that these cells are epithelial and not neuronal in origin, and are thought not to make 'connections' with the surrounding tissue. Currently, a randomized, sham-surgery controlled trial is ongoing.

Thus much more needs to be learned about the consequences of fetal or (hRPE) cell transplantation before these strategies can be considered viable/feasible options.

Future Directions

The entrance of molecular biology into the field of neural transplantation has led to exciting advances that greatly extend the ability to manipulate and generate cell lines that may be candidates for transplantation in PD and may ultimately supplant fetal grafting. Among the major new approaches to direct delivery of therapeutic agents into the central nervous system are:

- Infusion of neurotrophic factors
- *Ex vivo* and *in vivo* gene therapy
- Implantation of immortalized cells engineered to produce a specific protein.

■ Neurotrophic Factor Infusion

While theoretically attractive, restoration and maintenance of degenerating dopaminergic cell by infusion of neurotrophic factors has met with mixed success in early clinical trial. A large, multicenter, double-blind, placebo-controlled trial of intraventricular infusion of glial-cell derived neurotrophic factor showed no benefit at 8 months.[29] Autopsy results from one patient suggested that the neurotrophic factor was not reaching the target area, the striatum and substantia nigra. A subsequent open-label, clinical study that employed direct infusion of glial-cell derived neurotrophic into the putamen reported a 39% benefit in the "off" treatment UPDRS motor score in patients receiving up to 43.2 mg putamen per day of the neurotrophic factor.[30] However, a more rigorous randomized, placebo-controlled, trial was recently stopped due to lack of clinical efficacy, although the dose of glial-cell derived neurotrophic factor used in this study was significantly lower that in the earlier trial.[11]

■ *Ex Vivo* **Gene Therapy Using Autologous Cells**

In this hypothetical scenario, a PD patient's own cells (generally fibroblasts) are genetically modified to express tyrosine hydroxylase (TH), then are grafted into appropriate sites in the striatum to provide a local supply of levodopa at sites in the brain normally innervated by dopaminergic neurons.[31] The levodopa secreted by these cells may then be taken up by remaining neuronal and nonneuronal cells, converted to dopamine, and released in either a normally regulated or unregulated fashion. Grafted into MPTP-treated monkeys, autologous fibroblasts were found to express TH for up to 4 months.

■ *In Vivo* **Gene Transfer**

Various therapeutic transgenes have been delivered by various vectors in experimental models of PD. Proposed targets and strategies include the following:[32]

- Inhibition of apoptosis
- Transgene-mediated expression of glial cell line-derived neurotrophic factors
- Combined therapies of anti-apoptosis and GDNF
- Transgenes encoding enzymes involved in dopamine biosynthesis in the striatum
- Stem cells differentiated into functioning dopaminergic cells by genetic modification
- Transgene-mediated production of GABA in the STN.

Several vehicles have been used for in vivo transfer of cDNA sequences, including:[31]

- Herpes simplex viral vectors
- Adenoviral vectors (AAV)

- Direct plasmid DNA transfer
- Lentivirus vectors.

In an elegant experiment, the lentivirus vector was used to deliver the trophic factor GDNF into the striatum and substantia nigra of MPTP-treated monkeys.[33] Nigrostriatal activity was restored and motor function positively impacted. There were no serious adverse events.

A new trial utilizes infusion of recombinant AAV vectors expressing the two isoforms of the enzyme glutamic acid decarboxylase (GAD) into the subthalamic nucleus. The aim of this study is to promote GABA production by subthalamic glutaminergic cells, thereby changing the action of these neurons from excitatory to inhibitory.[34]

The optimal gene delivery vector remains in question and it is not known which proteins are required for adequate control of dopamine release. Thus, any cell that produces dopamine may also induce dyskinesias or psychiatric side effects unless dopamine release of such a cell is properly controlled. Another issue is the nonhuman genome that will be introduced into the human brain. Although all of these vectors (plasmids and viruses) have no known impact on mammalian cells, this cannot be excluded. Side effects may be caused by introduction of such genes. Therefore, the in vitro and in vivo experiments with gene transfer are interesting, but still very far from clinical application. Gene therapy with a beneficial trophic factor is much more promising, however the search continues for such a factor.

■ Implantation of Immortalized Cells

In this procedure, ventral mesencephalons are dissected from embryonic day 13 rats and dopaminergic cells are infected with the simian virus (SV 40) large T antigen, which renders them immortal at 33°C but permanently amitotic at 38° to 39°C. Once the cells are transfected, clonal lines of dopamine-producing cells can be established, resulting in a limitless supply of neuronal-like progenitors, all of which express TH and synthesize dopamine.

The immortalized cells may have some of the control mechanisms, but they also will contain a potentially harmful foreign genome. At present, it is not clear how much similarity there is with the endogenous dopaminergic neuron.

■ **Neuronal Precursor Cells**

In the central nervous system, there are two types of precursor cells:
- Omnipotent stem cells
- Pluripotent progenitor cells.

All of these cells have the ability to expand and to differentiate in various neurons or glial cells. Thus these cells are not genetically altered dividing cells that may provide an unlimited source of dopaminergic neurons. These cells can be easily obtained, cultured, and expanded from the embryonic and adult rodent and human brain. Our understanding of the regulation of such precursor cells is still limited. However, various investigators have been able to culture such precursor cells that contain a rather high percentage of dopaminergic neurons after differentiation.[35,36]

After transplantation in the dopamine-depleted rat brain, these cells are able to restore the dopaminergic deficit and compensate amphetamine-induced rotational behavior.[36] In the near future, it seems likely that factors and culture conditions will have been identified that allow a selective expansion of mesencephalic progenitor cells that, when transplanted into the human brain, will differentiate into dopaminergic neurons. Understanding the regulation of such immature neurons may also enable one to stimulate their proliferation in the adult brain, rendering transplantation unnecessary. Overall, these immature stem or progenitor cells, after appropriate selective proliferation, present the currently most promising source of "pure" dopaminergic neurons. These also have all the machinery to avoid excessive dopamine release.

REFERENCES

1. Verhagen L, O'Leary ST. The role of surgery in the treatment of motor complications. *Mov Disord.* 2005 Suppl DOI: 10.1002/mds.20480.

2. Tasker RR, Lang AE, Lozano AM. Pallidal and thalamic surgery for Parkinson's disease. *Exp Neurol.* 1997;144:35-40.

3. Hauser RA, Freeman TB, Olanow CW. Surgical therapies for Parkinson's disease. In: Kurlan R, ed. *Treatment of Movement Disorders.* Philadelphia, Pa: JB Lippincott Co; 1995:57-93.

4. Laitinen LV, Bergenheim AT, Hariz MI. Leksell's posteroventral pallidotomy in the treatment of Parkinson's disease. *J Neurosurg.* 1992;76:53-61.

5. Laitinen LV, Bergenheim AT, Hariz MI. Ventroposterolateral pallidotomy can abolish all parkinsonian symptoms. *Stereotact Funct Neurosurg.* 1992;58:14-21.

6. de Bie RM, de Haan RJ, Nijssen PC, et al. Unilateral pallidotomy in Parkinson's disease: a randomised, single-blind, multicenter trial. *Lancet.* 1999;354:1665-1669.

7. Fine J, Duff J, Chen R, et al. Long-term follow-up of unilateral pallidotomy in advanced Parkinson's disease. *N Engl J Med.* 2000;342:1708-1714.

8. Vitek JL, Bakay RA, Freeman A, et al. Randomized trial of pallidotomy versus medical therapy for Parkinson's disease. *Ann Neurol.* 2003;53:558-569.

9. Esselink RAJ, de Bie RMA, de Haan RJ, et al. Unilateral pallidotomy versus bilateral subthalamic nucleus stimulation in PD. A randomized trial. *Neurology.* 2004;62:201-207.

11

10. Goetz CG, Poewe W, Rascol O, Sampio C. Evidence-based medical review update: pharmacological and surgical treatments of Parkinson's disease: 2001-2004. *Mov Disord.* 2005;20: 523-539.

11. Walter BL, Vitek JL. Surgical treatment of Parkinson's disease. *Lancet Neurol.* 2004;3:719-728.

12. Diederich N, Goetz CG, Stebbins GT, et al. Blinded evaluation confirms long-term asymmetric effect of unilateral thalamotomy or subthalamotomy on tremor in Parkinson's disease. *Neurology.* 1992;42:1311-1314.

13. Koller W, Pahwa R, Busenbark K, et al. High-frequency unilateral thalamic stimulation in the treatment of essential and parkinsonian tremor. *Ann Neurol.* 1997;42:292-299.

14. Limousin P, Speelman JD, Gielen F, Janssens M. Multicentre European study of thalamic stimulation in parkinsonian and essential tremor. *J Neurol Neurosurg Psychiatry.* 1999;66: 289-296.

15. Lang AE, Lozano AM. Parkinson's disease. Second of two parts. *N Engl J Med.* 1998;339:1130-1143.

16. Limousin P, Krack P, Pollak P, et al. Electrical stimulation of the subthalamic nucleus in advanced Parkinson's disease. *N Engl J Med.* 1998;339:1105-1111.

17. Fraix V, Pollak P, Van Blercom N, et al. Effect of subthalamic nucleus stimulation on levodopa-induced dyskinesia in Parkinson's disease. *Neurology.* 2000;55:1921-1923.

18. Burchiel KJ, Anderson VC, Favre J, Hammerstad JP. Comparison of pallidal and subthalamic nucleus deep brain stimulation for advanced Parkinson's disease: results of a randomized, blinded pilot study. *Neurosurgery.* 1999;45:1375-1382.

19. Deep-Brain Stimulation for Parkinson's Disease Study Group. Deep-brain stimulation of the subthalamic nucleus or the pars interna of the globus pallidus in Parkinson's disease. *N Engl J Med.* 2001;345:956-963.

20. Katayama Y, Kasai M, Oshima H, et al. Subthalamic nucleus stimulation for Parkinson's disease: benefits observed in levodopa-intolerant patients. *J Neurosurg.* 2001;95:213-221.

21. Østergaard K, Sunde N, Dupont E. Effects of bilateral stimulation of the subthalamic nucleus in patients with severe Parkinson's disease and motor fluctuations. *Mov Disord.* 2002:17:693-700.

22. Jankovic J. Surgical treatment of Parkinson's disease. 11th Annual Course. A Comprehensive Review of Movement Disorders for the Clinical Practitioner. Aspen, Colo; August 3-6, 2001.

23. Lyons KE, Wilkinson SB, Overman J, Pahwa R. Surgical and hardware complications of subthalamic stimulation: a series of 160 procedures. *Neurology.* 2004;63:612-616.

24. Olanow CW, Freeman TB, Kordower JH. Transplantation strategies for Parkinson's disease. In: Watts RL, Koller WC, eds. *Movement Disorders: Neurologic Principles and Practice.* New York, NY: The McGraw-Hill Companies; 1997: 221-236.

25. Kordower JH, Goetz CG, Freeman TB, Olanow CW. Dopaminergic transplants in patients with Parkinson's disease: neuroanatomical correlates of clinical recovery. *Exp Neurol.* 1997;144:41-46.

26. Freed CR, Greene PE, Breeze RE, et al. Transplantation of embryonic dopamine neurons for severe Parkinson's disease. *N Engl J Med.* 2001;344:710-719.

27. Olanow CW, Goetz CG, Kordower JH, et al. A double-blind controlled trial of bilateral fetal nigral transplantation in Parkinson's disease. *Ann Neurol.* 2003;54:403-414.

28. Watts RL, Raiser CD, Stover NP, et al. Stereotactic intrastriatal implantation of human retinal pigment epithelial (hRPE) cells attached to gelatin microcarriers: a potential new cell therapy for Parkinson's disease. *J Neural Transm.* 2003;65(suppl):215-227.

29. Nutt JG, Burchiel KJ, Comella CL, et al. Randomized, double-blind trial of glial cell-derived neurotrophic factor (GDNF) in PD. *Neurology.* 2003;60:69-73.

30. Gill SS, Patel NK, Hotton GR, et al. Direct brain infusion of glial cell-derived neurotrophic factor in Parkinson disease. *Nat Med.* 2003;9:589-595.

31. Bankiewicz KS, Leff SE, Nagy D, et al. Practical aspects of the development of ex vivo and in vivo gene therapy for Parkinson's disease. *Exp Neurol.* 1997;144:147-156.

32. Burton EA, Glorioso JC, Fink DJ. Gene therapy progress and prospects: Parkinson's disease. *Gene Therapy.* 2003;10: 1721-1727.

33. Kordower JH, Emborg ME, Bloch J, et al. Neurodegeneration prevented by lentiviral vector delivery of GDNF in primate models of Parkinson's disease. *Science.* 2000;290:767-773.

34. During MJ, Kaplitt MG, Stern MB, Eidelberg D. Subthalamic GAD gene transfer in Parkinson disease patients who are candidates for deep brain stimulation. *Hum Gene Ther.* 2001; 12:1589-1591.

35. Ling ZD, Potter ED, Lipton JW, Carvey PM. Differentiation of mesencephalic progenitor cells into dopaminergic neurons by cytokines. *Exp Neurol.* 1998;149:411-423.

36. Studer L, Tabar V, McKay RD. Transplantation of expanded mesencephalic precursors leads to recovery in parkinsonian rats. *Nat Neurosci.* 1998;1:290-295.

INDEX

Note: Entries followed by "f" indicate figures; "t" tables.

Greek Characters

α-Adrenergic receptors, 193-195
α-Methyldopa, 83t
α-Synuclein, 23-29, 26t-27t, 54-57, 86
α-Synucleinopathies, 23-24
β-Amyloid fragments, 58
β-Blockers, 202
β-CIT, 86-87

Numbers

1-methyl-3-phenyl-1, 2, 3, 6-tetrahydropyridinen (MPTP)
   intoxication, 12t-13t, 14, 29-31, 55, 113-115
1-methyl-4-phenylpuridium ion (MPP+), 29-31, 55
5-Fluorouracil, 83t
26/20S proteasome, 53-54
1918-1928 pandemic, 80-81

Abilify, 83t, 188
Ablative procedures, 237-238. *See also* Surgical procedures.
Acquired immunodeficiency syndrome. *See* AIDS (acquired
   immunodeficiency syndrome).
Actigraphy, 198-199
Activities of Daily Living scale. *See* ADL (Activities of Daily
   Living) scale.
AD (Alzheimer's disease), 13t, 15, 23-24, 71t, 72-79
ADAS-cog scores, 186
ADL (Activities of Daily Living) scale, 88, 99t, 120-121
Aging, 23-24
Aging-related factors, 23-24
Agranulocytosis, 188
AIDS (acquired immunodeficiency syndrome), 12t-13t
Akathisia, 180-182, 181t, 183t, 202
Akinesia, 11
Alcohol use-related factors, 71t
Algorithm, progressive treatment, 104, 105f
Alien hand, 15
Alien limb phenomenon, 77-78
ALS (amyotrophic lateral sclerosis), 15
Alternative diagnoses, 63, 65t, 68t-69t
Alzheimer's disease. *See* AD (Alzheimer's disease).
Amantadine (Symmetrel), 105f, 107-112, 184-188, 202
Ambien, 199-200
American Academy of Neurology, 188

American Parkinson's Diseases Association, Inc., 218t-219t
American Speech-Language-Hearing Association, 225
Amiodarone, 83t
Amitriptyline, 82t
Amphotericin B, 83t
Amyotrophic lateral sclerosis. See ALS (amyotrophic lateral sclerosis).
Analgesics, 117
Ankle edema, 193-194
Anorectal dysfunction, 196-197
Anticholinergics, 85t, 106-107, 108t, 184-197, 202
Antidipressants, conventional, 189-191, 200
Antiemetics, 14
Antihypotensives, 195
Antiparkinson agents, listing of, 108t-111t
Antipsychotics, 14
Antiviral agents, 107, 112
Anxiety, 183t, 190-191
Apathy, 183t, 191-192
Apomorphine, 178-180, 178t
Apoptosis, 57-58. See also Pathogenesis.
Apraxia, 15
Archimedes spirals, 70f
Aricept, 185-186
Aripiprazole, 83t, 188
Arm X's and Y's, 221f-222f
Artane, 107, 108t
Associated disorders, 229-233, 233t
Ataxia, 14-15
Atropine-like drugs, 195-196
Atypical parkinsonism, 68t-69t
Autologous cells, 258
Autonomic disorders, 183t, 192-198
Azilect, 111t, 117-123, 119f, 121f-122f

Back thigh stretches, 220f
Ballism, 180
Baltimore Longitudinal Study of Aging, 23-24
Basal ganglia, 37-44, 38f-41f. See also under individual topics.
  GABA and, 40f-41f, 42-44
  GPi, 37, 38f, 40f-41f, 41-43
  intrathalmic nuclei, 38f, 39-40
  models of, 40f-41f
  SNr, 37-39, 38f-341f, 40-43
  striatum, 37, 38f
  subthalmic nucleus, 37, 38f
Basic topics. See Overviews and summaries.
Benzamide, 82t

12

12

12

12

12

12

12

12

12

12

12

12

12

12

12

12

12

12